# THE ULTIMATE TREADMILL WORKOUT

## Run Right, Hurt Less, and Burn More with **Treadmill Interval Training**

## David Siik
*Creator of Equinox's Precision Running*

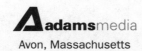

Avon, Massachusetts

## Testimonials

"I have been running all my life. Or, at least calling myself a runner. This year I met David, and I realized there is not just an art to running but a science too. His detailed instruction, his incredible energy, and overall great knowledge of the body have led me to a greater level of determination. I truly feel like I have broken new ground and reached new targets, in my forties! Who knew that was even possible? It's comforting to know the body can still work in such ways. With mindful instruction, we can achieve great results."

**—Naomi Watts, actress**

"Treadmill workouts will *never* be the same!"

**—Women's Health**

"There are many 'good' running coaches today, but David's skill and knowledge take it to a new echelon. He possesses that unique quality that enables him to both motivate and inspire people to greatness in running. Everyone needs to know about David Siik. If I was permitted only one fitness expert on my 'desert island,' David would be the one. He is the best of the best!"

**—Shay Mitchell, ABC Family's *Pretty Little Liars***

"David Siik is an amazing instructor, motivator, and expert trainer for those who love to run. I have played professional basketball in the NBA for the past 13 years. Having David as an instructor for the past couple years in my off-season has helped prepare me for each upcoming year. His training segments have a math and calculation, unique to his running method. The entire time he is energetically encouraging each runner to give their absolute best. At the end of each class I am thankful that I have a trainer that I can trust to make me a better athlete and better runner."

**—Jason Collins, NBA veteran**

# *Testimonials*

"David is to running what Tiger is to golf. He is simply the best at what he does. I was running on my own, doing the same steady pace and not seeing any results. When I discovered David's method of running, his perfectly programmed runs cut my workout time in half with amazing results, toning my legs, abs, and even my arms. I'm in better shape and I have fewer injuries than I ever have before. As a chiropractor, fewer injuries and longevity in maintaining a healthy lifestyle are important not only to me but for my patients as well. It's no wonder athletes and Hollywood's hottest bodies are in his classes everywhere. I have never been more excited for someone to write a book. It's about time!"

**—Dr. Carrie Schwartz, chiropractor**

Published by
Adams Media, a division of F+W Media, Inc.
57 Littlefield Street, Avon, MA 02322. U.S.A.
*www.adamsmedia.com*

ISBN 10: 1-4405-8929-1
ISBN 13: 978-1-4405-8929-4
eISBN 10: 1-4405-8930-5
eISBN 13: 978-1-4405-8930-0

Printed in the United States of America.

10   9   8   7   6   5   4   3   2   1

The information in this book should not be used for diagnosing or treating any health problem. Not all diet and exercise plans suit everyone. You should always consult a trained medical professional before starting a diet, taking any form of medication, or embarking on any fitness or weight-training program. The author and publisher disclaim any liability arising directly or indirectly from the use of this book.

Cover design by Sylvia McArdle.
Cover images © iStockphoto.com/YanC; Pali Rao; Brostock.
Author photo by Ian Maddox.

*This book is available at quantity discounts for bulk purchases.*
*For information, please call 1-800-289-0963.*

# CONTENTS

Introduction . . . 7

## Part One: MASTERING THE TREADMILL . . . 13

Chapter 1: THE BITE METHOD . . . 15

Chapter 2: TREADMILL BASICS . . . 23

Chapter 3: INCLINE—YOUR FRENEMY! . . . 31

Chapter 4: SPEED—SMART IS THE NEW FAST . . . 41

Chapter 5: DURATION—TOO SHORT VS. TOO LONG . . . 51

Chapter 6: RECOVERY—NOT ALWAYS EASY . . . 57

Chapter 7: FORM—CRITICAL MISTAKES ON THE TREADMILL . . . 65

Chapter 8: INJURIES AND LIMITATIONS . . . 73

Chapter 9: EARN IT! . . . 81

## Part Two: THE TREADMILL WORKOUT . . . 83

Chapter 10: THE WORKOUTS . . . 85

Chapter 11: THREE-WEEK KICK-START . . . 89

Chapter 12: THE SIX-WEEK RUNNING REVOLUTION . . . 129

Appendix A: DIET AND HEALTH . . . 215

Appendix B: TREADMILL TROUBLESHOOTING . . . 219

# RUN SMART. HURT LESS. BURN MORE.

I'm going to tell you one of the greatest secrets in fitness—nothing, and I mean nothing, is ever going to replace the run. It is the most natural, effective, and guaranteed way to change your body and your life. You can spend the rest of your days avoiding this reality. You can empty your wallet every day seeking out the newest trend, the shortcut, or the inflated promise of results without work. You can look yourself in the mirror every morning and convince yourself you're going to find an easier way to lose that weight or strengthen your body. Or, you can look yourself in the mirror, take a deep breath, and consider putting the word *work* back in your workout. You can make the choice to embark on what is real, what works, and what human beings have been designed to do for over 2.5 million years. You were born with attributes so specific for running that if you didn't have them, the act of running would be nearly impossible. Take our glutes for example: Their very proportion, size, and placement give us power when we sprint; we can't sprint without them! Improving your speed work allows your glutes to do exactly what they were designed to do. Give them the right environment, and in no time you'll see a higher, tighter, rounder booty, and there isn't a human being on this planet who doesn't want that. It's not just your glutes either. Daniel Lieberman, an evolutionary biologist from Harvard, reminds us that even the length of our toes is specific to our running design. Animals that are designed to run *must* have short digits on their feet in order to not break them with the force of running. Cheetahs have tiny toes and are one of the fastest animals on the planet, while the orangutan's lanky toes render it nearly incapable of running. So the next time you say, "Oh, I'm not a runner," then please, by all means, start walking on your long-fingered hands. Forget about your abs, let the belly hang out, and forget about your ass, 'cause you will definitely not need that anymore. Take some pride, accept how you were made, and celebrate that you were designed with the sleek and beautiful attributes of a cheetah and not an orangutan. It is almost ironic that the very changes most of us want to make in our bodies, the flatter stomach, the nicer butt, the lean, strong body, are all side effects of doing the most natural locomotion mankind has ever known, simply running.

If a healthier, sexier body isn't enough to motivate you, let me tell you a little something you didn't know about running. How would you like to reduce the risk of death from Alzheimer's by 40%? I sure the hell would, and guess what, it's not from eating kale or drinking coconut water—it is from running! The results of an extensive study conducted at the Lawrence Berkeley National Laboratory in California first published in 2014 showed this risk reduction in participants who ran an average of 15 miles per week. It is no coincidence that this is the average mileage per week you will be hitting with the workouts in the book. But, you have to make the choice to do the work.

The treadmill is the most sold fitness machine in the world, surpassing $1 billion in sales in 2014. The reason for this is simple. No other machine comes close to helping you achieve faster and more dramatic results. Again, it works. Machines such as the elliptical, the stair stepper, and that weird machine (you have no idea what it does) all do one thing very well: They reduce overall workload compared to running. And although no one wants you to know this, that is exactly what they are designed to do. These machines lack the incredible health benefits and the untouchable fat-burning results of running. The treadmill is the *only* machine that can give you the combined benefits of all those machines, plus the life-changing ones they cannot. And furthermore, it is the only machine that translates to your everyday life. You aren't likely to enter the New York City Elliptical Marathon anytime soon! If you are ready for something real, I can help you feel more alive, more excited, and more powerful than you ever have in your life. I can help you lose weight fast and finally see the lean, strong body you have always wanted. And I can show you how to do all of this in an exciting, balanced, and effective way. If you don't already, you will come to love running. Running is the healthiest addiction you can have. This book is not a shortcut, and I will not promise you that it is the easiest workout. I can promise you, however, that it works.

*The Ultimate Treadmill Workout* is designed to do three things. First, it will show you how to run on the treadmill in the safest and most effective way. Second, with its signature formula and flow, it will provide you with the most incredible interval experience you have ever had on a treadmill. You can now do the same workouts reserved for fitness classes, celebrities, and world-class athletes. You will become so engaged in your workouts that you won't believe just how fun and interesting the treadmill can actually be. And last, you will burn more fat with less pain than you ever thought was possible.

I see the person who needs this book in every walk of life. It's you and it's me. It's the person with a treadmill in the basement, collecting dust and being used as a clothing rack. It's the everyday gym-goer, standing on a treadmill, pushing Start, looking lost and bored for a few minutes, then wandering off to see if the elliptical or bike is any more exciting. It's the hard-core studio class participant, pounding away to a great beat and sexy lighting, wondering if this is really the best way to do things. And yes, it's even you, outdoor runner, my old friend, already rolling your eyes at the very thought of a treadmill book. I see all of you, every day of my life. And knowing that you didn't have access to an all-in-one guide for using the treadmill in today's world, I decided to write it for you.

Over a decade ago I began exploring treadmill running and workouts. I had recently come off a successful and fulfilling career as a college 800-meter sprinter, and I was hungry to explore new running adventures and workouts. The more I explored, the more I discovered there was a gaping hole in the world of running. For too long, everyone had underestimated the value of proper treadmill training. As treadmill classes began popping up, even a decade ago, I knew we were experiencing the rise of the treadmill era—the rise of the machines. I assure you, if you haven't noticed yet, that time has arrived. Technology and innovation have unleashed treadmill running like never before. I also realized a huge mistake brewing in this trend, the lack of information. As happens so often in health and fitness, the products, ideas, and trends grow out of an obsession to burn fat, and burn it fast. Herein lies the entire reason I want you to have this book. You see, burning fat should never be the focus of a running program; it is simply an incredible side effect. If you create a treadmill workout based only on the burn, you gut it of the balancing principles of running science, and the very spirit of the running experience. You also create an environment that far too often leads to injury, frustration, and ultimately the end of your relationship with running. This is the undeniable truth about running: You're going to burn fat, a lot of it. But you have to do it right, no matter if you're on the street or on the treadmill. I do believe this is largely why the outdoor-running community has never really fully embraced this treadmill-running trend, because it seems artificial, lacking in running science and the rich and complex history of running. So, what if we did inject the intelligent and emotional sport of outdoor running into a method designed specifically for the treadmill? The result: a comprehensive running program that safely produces the results and spirit of the run, but does so with the comfort, technology, and efficiency of the treadmill. It's track practice on a treadmill.

My entire career is coaching treadmill workouts and innovating better ways to experience the runner's high on the machine. This book is written by a real runner, but more importantly, by someone who lives and breathes all things "treadmill." Years of research, testing, and coaching have led me to develop the Balanced Interval Training Experience, the BITE method. It is a product of 25 years of experience as a competitive runner, a constant thirst for science, and a deeply sentimental and compassionate approach to running. This new option in interval training is designed to maximize the burn and eliminate the pain when using a treadmill, which is an innovation in itself. It is a revolutionary formula that combines running science with the unique capabilities of the treadmill to create a safe, honest, electrifying, and above all else, extremely effective workout. With this book, I want you to know it's okay to be in love with something so classic, so affective, and so natural as the run. But not just any run. A new running method that takes your natural instincts, crosses them with the best science and research on running, and challenges you to meet—and exceed—your fitness goals, whether you are a seasoned marathoner or about to try on running sneakers for the first time. With the information and carefully calibrated treadmill workouts in this book, everything old is new again.

You see, running is unlike anything else in fitness. I have traveled all over the country giving lectures and trainings on running, and I always remind people of this very important truth: If you strip away everything, every bicycle, stair stepper, elliptical, dumbbell, jump rope, every gadget or gimmick you have sitting in a box in your garage, every class you have ever taken, and everything you have ever learned about fitness, the only thing you will have left in the end is the run. It is the single seed that sprouted the entire forest of fitness. Over 2.5 million years old, running is ingrained in the DNA of what makes us human beings. The ability to walk and run makes us powerful and limitless. We have learned a great deal about this ability, and we should demand this information be transferred from the forest to the treadmill. And so, I created a method that successfully bridges this gap and transfers this information for the new age of urban running.

Whether you are a treadmill devotee with your own home model, or walk by it in the gym without a second glance, or you already take a treadmill class, this book will completely change how you look at the experience. Filled with life-changing workouts, never-before-shared tips, and a motivational kick in the pants, this is truly the only treadmill-running book you will ever need. And because running is so personal and intensely emotional I will not only show you how; I will tell you why. I will not shy away from sharing my greatest victories, the failures, the trips and falls, and the love and losses I've experienced in my own journey in becoming the running coach I am today.

*The Ultimate Treadmill Workout* will not only teach you a better way to run, it will inspire you and be the ultimate reminder that the run is the oldest, truest, and most loyal companion you will ever have in your quest for health and fitness. Running has always been and will always be. No more excuses, no more gadgets, no more shortcuts. It's time to dust off that treadmill and get back to what works. With the help of this book you will finally have the opportunity to master your greatest running potential. And you will do this with the help of one of the greatest innovations in human history, the treadmill. It's time for you to start running smart, hurting less, and burning more. It's time to return to the run. So take a deep breath, make the choice to do this work, and get ready to set your body and spirit on fire!

# PART ONE

# MASTERING THE TREADMILL

## Chapter 1

# THE BITE METHOD

The best method for treadmill training is the one that produces the best results in the least amount of time, with the least amount of impact on the body. It is the perfect recipe for the new age of treadmill training. You hear a lot about fat-burning results and quick workouts, but you have to have them *and* be able to have longevity in running and fitness. I'm giving you a way to do all this without trashing your body.

This book introduces the first comprehensive method specifically engineered for the treadmill workout experience. This method tackles the most important truth about running: It doesn't matter where you do it, what technology you use, or even what new buzz-worthy studio you go to—what will always matter most is the content and design of your run.

The quality of a run is the single most important element of treadmill training. The lights, the music, the screaming coach on the microphone, the cool new app—all of that is great, but it will never be more valuable than the quality of the run itself. The most empowering and effective method of treadmill running is the one that has the single goal of creating the prefect run. The balanced formula and set of guidelines in this book is the closest I have ever come to finding that "perfect run." It will allow you to become a stronger runner, experience the greatest calorie burn, bring life and meaning into your workout, and minimize the cost to your body. Let everyone else worry about distractions. You worry about the smart work that will last you for the rest of your life.

People hesitate to run on a treadmill for four reasons:

1. They don't want to do the work.
2. They are concerned that it might not be good for their joints.
3. They feel unsteady or dizzy on the treadmill.
4. They simply don't know what to do and are bored.

On the flip side, there is an increasing number of people flocking to treadmill running, but they are plagued with injuries or plateaus. We will address and eliminate all of these concerns in this book, but regardless of the reason, the new running method you are about to be introduced to is the secret recipe that will turn any hesitation into excitement. And the results will be incredible. It is the same workout method I have coached to A-list celebrities, pregnant women, professional athletes, 80-year-olds, and 20-year-old track-and-field stars. You don't have to be a running expert or even an experienced runner to allow this new method to change your body, your attitude, and ultimately, your life.

## The Balanced Interval Training Experience—BITE

### BITE the Bullet

How does the BITE method work? BITE finds the optimal middle ground between sprinting and distance training. It works by challenging your body to use the four essential treadmill training elements in a newly prescribed way:

1. Interval: Mathematically formulated bursts of running with the perfect variations in intensity.
2. Speed: A first-ever balancing speed concept to use the right speed to enhance the other elements in a safer and more effective way.
3. Incline: A new science-based scale of adding the best amount of hill work with limits on steepness versus speed.

4. Recovery: An entirely new outlook on how you *should* be resting between interval work.

By using a unique cycle of sprinting and endurance intervals, BITE will give you the most comprehensive treadmill workout with incredible results—as long as you're willing to bite the bullet and put in the work.

---

The BITE method uses a revolutionary formula to create a safer, more balanced, and attainable approach to achieving the same mega-burn as any other form of interval training, but with the least amount of impact. This more comprehensive approach has created guidelines and awareness that are changing the landscape of how we run on treadmills, and is the first and only treadmill method with a complete system of balancing all the principles of running. This creates a safer sweat.

The most important difference in this new running program is not the amount of work you do, but rather the balance in how you do it. That is the real game-changer. Even novice runners are surprised by how much they can do, and how good it can feel.

There are basically two forms of treadmill workouts:

1. High-intensity interval training (HIIT)
2. Steady-state cardio

You might be surprised to know that neither of these forms of treadmill running is actually a running program. There is no such thing. They are a broad-based fitness and cardiovascular concept of working out, based largely on heart rate. There are HIIT cycling workouts, lifting workouts, swimming, jumping rope—you name it, it can fit into this model. And this is exactly where I found the greatest opportunity to help treadmill users. Someone needed to create an actual running program, based on running, for runners. A program that takes decades of scientific research, years of personal experience, observation, testing, and treadmill coaching and combines them to create the most powerful treadmill workout imaginable. Wanting this for you, I created this new method. It is, in essence, an interval-training model exclusively for treadmill workouts. It adopts the best benefits from both HIIT and steady-state cardio, but does so with a running formula rich with principles, guidelines, and limits unique to running that do not currently exist in the broader definition of HIIT or steady-state cardio. And so the BITE method was born. It is a smart, smooth, balance-driven middle ground between the other forms of treadmill training. It is this balanced approach that creates what I call TreadFlow, a progression of work, creating one of the smoothest and most effective treadmill workouts you will ever experience.

If this all sounds complicated, let me show you how different treadmill workouts compare. Understanding this is extremely useful not only when you attempt the workouts in this book, but also when you find yourself trying out the newest treadmill class. And remember, the BITE method isn't designed to compete with other running programs. It is rooted in science and common-sense running information, so that above all else, it is designed to make you a more educated runner. Like everything in life, knowledge is the most empowering tool you can ever have. Let's start by looking at the "work" you do when you do intervals. If you look at intervals with an effort scale of 1–5, it becomes easy to see how the two common running workouts compare with BITE, and how this new method helps you reach the same goal, with less time and physical stress on your body, and in a much more interesting way.

### HIIT (Sprint)

HIIT adopts the idea of using difficult intervals with easier recoveries, and has become one of the most popular weight-loss tools in recent years. The idea of high-intensity intervals has spread far and wide throughout the fitness industry. And although I don't deny the effectiveness in using this method to burn fat, I am deeply concerned when it is mistaken for a running program or method. If you are going to use the treadmill to become a better runner, burn fat, and become stronger, it is imperative that you have a balanced and comprehensive plan so that it's not just effective, but also safe and sustainable. Let's look at the balance of work using a scale of 1–5. A 1 would be a light effort; think a light jog of 4 mph. A 5 would be a maximum effort and sprint, likely over 9 mph. On the 1–5 scale, hitting maximum burns of 5 all the time means you are also putting the maximum impact and force on the body, all the time.

And I can assure you if this is all you do, you will burn out, or worse, deal with unnecessary injuries, aches, and pains.

$$5 + 5 = 10$$

### Steady-State Cardio (Distance)

Often steady-state cardio is seen as a form of distance running. It most often consists of maintaining a constant average pace over multiple miles or time without recovery periods. On the 1–5 scale you can see how you'll need to spend significantly more time hitting steady 1s to achieve the same results. I believe this is the least effective way to do a treadmill workout, largely because of the lack of change, which contributes to the biggest problem people have on a treadmill—boredom. It has also been shown to be the least effective way of running to burn fat. I never recommend, nor do most running coaches, using distance training like marathon training for fat loss. Distance training is critical in conquering your first marathon or triathlon. It serves a wonderful and powerful purpose in preparing for long races or enjoying a long, beautiful trail run, but it isn't ever going to be your most efficient use of time for fat burning.

$$1 + 1 + 1 + 1 + 1 + 1 + 1 + 1 + 1 + 1 = 10$$

### BITE

The BITE method replaces the mindless miles with engaging intervals. Unlike HIIT, this method introduces an exclusive and specific set of guidelines and principles that are designed *only* for the treadmill workout experience. It is intense interval training, so you'll be sure to burn fat. But because it comes with a unique formula of balance, it reduces the excessive wear and tear on the body. This will leave you not only more fit, but also feeling great from head to toe for years to come. The smoothness of the BITE method is something everyone feels immediately. Like everything in fitness, there is a price to be paid for disregarding balance, an element crucial to healthy running. Because the BITE method blends the strength-training benefits of sprint training with the endurance benefits of distance running, the method naturally strikes an intricate middle ground between sprint training (HIIT) and steady state (distance), giving way to a new hybrid form of interval training. Uniquely, this is the only method to have a signature mathematical value system of increasing effort gradually and specifically for the perfect burn. This value system is revealed for you in each of the variable chapters—incline, speed, duration, and recovery. Put together, these variables create the ultimate TreadFlow.

## TreadFlow

*TreadFlow* is the term I use for the unique rhythm of each run. The balancing of math and the chain reaction that progresses interval to interval are what create this signature flow. It's what gives each workout a smooth build in effort. You may not always understand the formula built into each workout, but your body is guaranteed to feel the "flow."

On the 1–5 scale you can see the work isn't reduced, but rather shifted and reformulated.

$$1 + 2 + 3 + 4 = 10$$

Looking at all the models together is a great way to compare them.

### HIIT (Sprint)
$$5 + 5 = 10$$

### Steady-State Cardio (Distance)
$$1 + 1 + 1 + 1 + 1 + 1 + 1 + 1 + 1 + 1 = 10$$

### BITE

1 + 2 + 3 + 4 = 10

Using the BITE system, you will go fast, but not too fast. You will still recover, but at a calculated amount.

As a more complete, balanced approach to high-intensity interval training, BITE relies on the integrity of a formula founded on a well-developed set of guidelines with checks and balances. This takes away the guesswork and reduces the risk of injury due to uninformed training. The systematic and mathematical nature of the interval creates workouts that are challenging and extremely interesting. You will feel and come to love the flow.

In the following chapters, I will share these unique guidelines, covering all major components of any treadmill workout. Whether you are doing a workout from this book at home or you are in a treadmill class, you will be empowered with the knowledge to run smarter. Here are some of the important things you will learn in the following chapters regarding the components of the BITE method:

- How to apply the perfect amount of incline to the proper speed
- How to increase speed safely and effectively
- The perfect interval length
- The importance of active recovery

Finally, you can begin doing interval training based on the science of running and the experience of actual runners, each facet complementing and reinforcing the other. It is specific and calculated, guiding you not only to great success, but most importantly, to sustainable success. Do sprint work on the track, do distance runs on the trail, and do BITE running on the treadmill. This method has become my personal "running fountain of youth," keeping me incredibly fit, energized, and most importantly, injury-free. It has been an emotional journey of mistakes and victories, experiment and discovery. *The Ultimate Treadmill Workout*'s transformative ability is the result of using this new, balanced approach and a more sustainable way to run on the treadmill. This method will set your body free and your spirit ablaze, leaving you excited, motivated, and above all, stronger than you ever thought possible.

## KEY POINTS FROM CHAPTER 1

- The BITE method is the most balanced approach to treadmill interval training.

- BITE workouts create a fun and engaging TreadFlow for a smooth run.

- BITE is a new method for reducing the wear and tear and aches and pains, without sacrificing any of the fat burn.

- BITE finds a middle ground between distance training and sprint training.

## Chapter 2

# TREADMILL BASICS

All over the world people are flocking to the treadmill like never before. You may have heard the buzz about treadmill classes and studios, or you may have run across one of the many apps designed for treadmill workouts. Treadmill technology and innovation have collided with our need to get back to the basics of what really works. Still, many people feel disdain for the treadmill—in fact, you may be one of them. The number-one reason people avoid the treadmill is that they don't know what to do once they get on it. Others feel bored or nervous it's not good for them, or are simply avoiding putting in the "work." I understand each of these reactions. I've built a career helping people break through those feelings. By the end of this book, you will not only have an entirely new perspective on the treadmill, but you will actually begin to enjoy it as well. Ultimately, you will find one of the fastest, truest, safest ways to a better body and healthier life.

Before you even begin this journey of indoor running, you need to know how this machine can work for you. There are four unbeatable benefits you can expect to experience from treadmill running. No other environment for running offers these essential benefits:

1. Time efficiency
2. Less joint impact
3. Less environmental stress
4. Data collection

Let's take a look at what each of these perks can offer you in your workout.

### More Work, Less Time

Interval running outside can be challenging, time consuming, and difficult to plan. The wonderful thing about the treadmill is that it's a giant computer, capable of giving you a reliable and efficient workout, when you want it and how you want it. The treadmill is also incapable of lying to you. It is a truly honest machine. Once you input a speed and incline, the machine takes over the responsibility of holding you accountable. You *will* do more work, in less time, and see much faster results.

We live busy lives, and let's be honest, we all want the biggest bang for our minutes in the gym. For me, this is arguably the greatest reason I use the treadmill. Rather than a shortcut, it's just real work done in a short amount of time. Few types of cardio will allow you to burn as many calories per minute as running, and with the great tools the treadmill offers, it ramps up that burn to an incredible full-body workout. The majority of the workouts in this book are less than 30 minutes, and although that may seem like a long time to be on a treadmill, the amount of work you do in that time is immense. The treadmill is the perfect machine to get you in and get you out, so you can spend a little more time doing the other things in life you'd rather be doing!

### Turn the TV Off!

If the treadmill is completely new to you, it can seem a bit overwhelming to know which one is the best for you or even how to use the machine. Don't worry; if you can use a cell phone, you can learn to use any treadmill. The fastest-evolving component of the treadmill is the monitor. Most monitors display speed, incline, mileage, time, and sometimes metrics like heart rate or calories. If you are choosing a treadmill at your gym I recommend that you stay clear of ones with a TV built into the monitor, or if yours has a TV, *turn it off*. Watching TV is as big of a distraction as sending e-mails in the middle of your workout. Don't do it. You will get so much more work done so much faster if you focus only on your workout. Unless the machine is brand new, you likely won't need to set anything like mph or kph. Just step on, turn the machine on, and begin warming up.

After you get your treadmill moving it's important to familiarize yourself with the buttons. Most treadmills have speed controls on the right-hand side and incline controls on the left. The placement of the buttons varies greatly, and new treadmills often have them in two locations, on a touch screen and on the treadmill itself. Either way, familiarize yourself with the locations of the controls.

Get comfortable with the treadmill before you start sprinting. Accidents do happen, but it's almost always user error. If you are new to treadmills or are getting on an unfamiliar treadmill, practice stepping off onto the side rails (small platforms on each side of the belt) and back on while walking. If you ever get caught up or something goes wrong, simply stepping off to the sides is the quickest, safest way to avoid an injury. Every treadmill has a safety "kill" switch, and although people rarely if ever use them, know that it is there for your use. Most of them clip onto your clothing so that if you do happen to stumble it will immediately stop the belt. Take a deep breath and don't worry. Of the thousands of runners I have coached on treadmills I have only ever seen two falls, both of which were brought on by things the runners should not have been doing on a treadmill.

### The Ultimate Low-Impact Surface

Today's treadmills are not only efficient but also kinder to the joints. Hard surfaces such as sidewalks and streets do little to absorb shock. Concrete, one of the hardest surfaces to run on, is unfortunately *everywhere*. The time and distance it takes for many of us to travel to a knee-friendly environment is simply time in our weeks we do not have. The treadmill creates a shock-absorbing environment in your own home, or in your local gym. The treadmill gives you the perfect opportunity to stop hitting the pavement and work on becoming a stronger, healthier runner.

Although every treadmill will provide a lower-impact surface than the sidewalk, there are many different treadmills on the market. Nearly every treadmill has a traditional belt system. When you are choosing a treadmill in the gym, you want to make sure the treadmill is stable, first and foremost. There are feet adjustments on many treadmills to make sure they are level to the ground, and sometimes they are off a bit. If you start walking on the treadmill and you immediately feel the treadmill wobbling from side to side, I recommend trying a different treadmill. If you are dusting off your good old treadmill at home, test it out and if it feels like it is wobbling when you get moving, you may need to adjust the feet, or you may need to put it on a flatter, more stable surface. When you are working out on a treadmill it is important that it is straight and sturdy. The ground is already moving underneath you, so the last thing you need is it moving from side to side as well as front to back. It's like that annoying table leg at a restaurant, except putting some sugar packets under a treadmill leg isn't likely to help.

If you are in the market to purchase a new treadmill, which I think is a great investment, the best thing you can do is go to a store and test them out. Most fitness supply stores that sell treadmills will have display models to test out. Again, the number-one thing I tell people to look out for is sturdiness. If it feels shaky and wobbly, try something else. The moment you get on a solid, sturdy treadmill, you'll know immediately. Keep in mind also, treadmills range greatly in price, and you really do get what you pay for. The industry builds treadmills based on usage. A cheaper treadmill doesn't necessarily mean it's cheaply made, but rather it is intentionally void of certain components not necessary for some people's use. If you know you are never going to be sprinting over 10 mph, you don't need a treadmill with a motor that revs up the belt to 15 mph. Treadmill companies offer models with lower-cost motors that will suit your needs, and cost you less. Again, the feel of a treadmill is the best way to choose the right one. People often tell me, "David, I'm not experienced enough to know how it should feel." But they always come back to me astounded by how different every treadmill feels, and like a good pair of shoes, how there is one that fits just right.

One thing I tell people is not to spend too much time stressing over fancy add-ons. If two treadmills both feel great and one is significantly more expensive because it has a built-in misting fan and 15 cup holders, you should save yourself a buck and go with the quality one that is void of the things you don't really need. If you are planning on using a treadmill a lot and have other family members who will be using it as well, I recommend spending a little more money for a treadmill that is closer to a commercial scale. They are a bit pricier, but they are built to handle many users and many miles. Again, you get what you pay for in a treadmill. Finally, check warranty and user ratings. It's a significant purchase, and customers are happy to rate and comment on their satisfaction. You'll learn a lot about the machine that way, and it's worth the investigation. Warranties are pretty standard across the board, but it's smart to compare them, because like all machines, a treadmill will someday need some maintenance.

Regardless of the treadmill you get on, or choose to purchase, you are taking a positive step in the right direction. It is also important to note that although the treadmill allows for only a little less impact on the joints, that difference is important to your overall health. This is the great benefit of running. Done right, it will help you maintain strong bones and healthy joints as you age. Science has always been on the side of maintaining a healthy amount of impact on our joints throughout our lives. For most people it's not that running is bad for your knees, it's that *not* running is bad for your knees. Put that on a T-shirt!

One only has to put aside rumors and look at statistics to be reminded of the benefits of running. Studies, including the massive study done by the Lawrence Berkeley National Laboratory, found a significant reduction in osteoarthritis and hip replacement in runners compared to walkers (though this doesn't mean you won't also see benefits from interval training if you are a walker). Study after study shows that runners maintain higher bone mass density as they age. Even among swimmers and cyclists, runners are the true champs of strong, healthy bones. I could write an entire book providing proof that running is actually essential for optimal health as you age. Too much running or improper running, like everything else in life, can be hard on the body. But the right amount, done the right way, as recommended in this book, can be one of the best things you ever do for your body, for now and for the long haul. The excuse that running is bad for you has long been put to rest in the medical community, and it's time for anyone else still using excuses to do the same.

### Healthy Skin, Clean Lungs

Sun damage is one of the harshest environmental factors that runners must deal with when running outdoors. Every year, more and more compelling research and information come out, warning us to limit our sun exposure. A runner's skin can take a beating from the elements over the years, and you don't have to endure that beating just to become a better runner or to look and feel healthier. I encourage everyone to enjoy running in the great outdoors. This book is not designed to persuade people to stop running outdoors, but to give a positive and worthwhile experience for those who choose or need to use the treadmill. Running outside is important, but it doesn't need to be the only place you run, and frankly it isn't always the best place to learn to become a better runner. If you are serious about making a change and letting running help you make that change, balancing that weekend trail run with a muscle-toning, calorie-destroying treadmill workout is one of the best decisions you could ever make. Again, you have to make the choice to do this work.

Temperature is also something every runner must consider at some point. Do I wear a hat? Do I wear thermal pants or a jacket? And if you're from northern Michigan like me, do I wear a ski mask, scarf, snowmobile suit, hand warmers, and snow shoes in order to brave the below-zero winter months? And what time? Is it better to run in the cool mornings of summer or the heat of the afternoon? Cold, dry, wintery conditions can often lead to injuries, more damaged skin, and the inability to maximize your potential. Pollution, particularly carbon monoxide (CO), doesn't fully combust when it's cold; it sits lower to the ground and goes right into your lungs. Many people don't realize they are actually breathing heavier pollutants in the cold winter months than the hot muggy summers. Running indoors, especially for those with asthma or other breathing conditions, creates a much safer, less stressful experience in running. And let's not forget about the many hazards of slippery roads. Falling on your ass is a rite of passage in northern Michigan, but it need not happen during your run.

It's not just cold winter months that make the treadmill a logical choice. Hot summer air can be equally hard on the body. Prolonged exposure to heat, which creates an elevated body temperature, can wreak havoc on the cells of your body. Running in extreme heat is also dangerous, especially for an inexperienced runner. Heat stroke is a very real thing. I know firsthand, and it isn't pleasant—and it certainly isn't worth it. Again, the treadmill makes its case. Running on a treadmill indoors is kind of like living in Southern California, with its predictably pleasant weather, all the time. Whether you are running in a temperature-perfect gym or setting just the right temperature in your home, eliminating that environmental stress alone can allow you to better focus on the work, change the way you feel, and equally as important, change the way you look.

### *Tracking Your Success*

We live in the digital age, where data is more available, recordable, and usable than ever before. This is good for runners. The best results in running performance come with the precise execution of the workout. It is the treadmill itself that allows for such precision. This is exactly why I decided to work with the renowned Equinox fitness clubs to create the world's best and only method-based treadmill class, Precision Running. Equinox is a true leader in innovation and dedication to cutting-edge, content-driven group fitness classes, so it was a perfect place to introduce the method of running described in this book. The treadmill's data-gathering capabilities are essential to utilizing precise running science. Remember, the treadmill is a giant computer. It doesn't have an opinion on how fast, how steep, or how far you go. It tells you exactly what you are doing, to the second, to the 0.5% grade, to the tenth of a mile per hour. This information is what allowed me to create a formula so rich with content and endless capabilities. The treadmill also allows you to monitor your achievements and set goals for greatness. There is no running experience that can give you that much data all at your fingertips. If you are using or have purchased a new treadmill, chances are you have a large digital display screen, perhaps even a touch screen. Take your time getting used to the monitor—play with it, and learn what display options it has. Many treadmills allow you to input one to three set interval speeds for a quick speed-up, so instead of holding down the plus button for speed you have a one-push button for a set speed. There are also many display options to choose from, and I always recommend you choose the one that has the biggest, clearest image of a running clock. It will be helpful in keeping track of your timing. For those of you in the market for a treadmill and who enjoy monitoring results, be sure to look into treadmills with monitors that have Wi-Fi capabilities and connectors to your smartphone. The next several years are going to see some incredible advances in running-data collection and usage, so make sure your treadmill will be ready to connect to all these great products coming out.

I'm not here to convince you to use the treadmill; I am here to help you unlock the best way to use it and give you the best workouts you have ever had on the treadmill. Confidence, however, is the key to success in any fitness program. Be confident that the treadmill is one of the greatest opportunities to strengthen your relationship with running and to experience real change.

## KEY POINTS FROM CHAPTER 2

- You'll do the largest amount of work in the smallest amount of time.

- Familiarize yourself with the capabilities of the monitor and avoid watching TV.

- Treadmills provide a lower-impact surface upon which to do the work.

- Choose a treadmill that is even and stable on the floor.

- Running indoors will reduce environmental stress on your skin and your lungs.

- The treadmill is a computer. It will keep you more honest than almost any other machine in the world. It will allow you to see real progress and plan goals with laser precision.

## Chapter 3

# INCLINE—YOUR FRENEMY!

*Gravity is a bitch. And I'm not talking about wrinkles.*

*My respect for "inclines" started a long time ago, on a hot day in August of 2002. The old Grand Valley State University ski hill near Grand Rapids, Michigan, is a formidable incline, unforgiving and seemingly endless. Running up the horrible, grassy, uneven, and often muddy hill that my university track team used for preseason conditioning is the closest I've ever come to puking from exercising. There was nothing I hated and loved more at the same time. We ran it in groups, and we ran it fast, over and over until our quads caught fire. And even though I always finished the workout, the hill always won, and years later I realized it always will.*

*But incline can make you incredibly strong, and it can burn a lot of calories. From an appearance standpoint, inclines magnify the work on your butt and your thighs, helping lift and shape your glutes and creating amazing definition in your thighs. I always tell people, the right amount of incline will give you a "little tiny waist and nice round base." Every Monday in August, for 4 years, the ski hill left me a pale, gasping, twitching pile of a runner. I'll never forget looking up at that hill for the first time through the rose-tinted lenses of my 18-year-old naiveté and thinking, No big deal. The coaches I barely knew were finally going to see me run. I shook out my hands and got ready to show the hill I was fearless. Little did I know the hill was laughing and I was the joke.*

*Over a decade later I found myself on a treadmill climbing another hill. It was many years and many miles from that old ski hill at my university. As I was zipping up the steep incline, I was suddenly transported back to that ski hill I thought I had escaped. I gritted my teeth and hammered away, clinging to the faintest semblance of decent running form. I could smell the long, dry grass and hear the buzzing of grasshoppers; I remembered every detail of that hill. And then I caught a glimpse of myself in the mirror. And like a lightning bolt I was ripped from the memory and back to reality. I stepped onto the sides of the treadmill, staring at my slumped body in the mirror. I couldn't breathe, my back hurt, and something felt off in one of my knees. I stared hard at myself wondering,* Where did the last 10 years go? *It was at that moment I realized my body was no longer 18 years old, I no longer had a coach to impress, and there was no competitor to beat. Suddenly a revelation took hold—something else had to change. I wasn't running to beat someone; I was running to stay healthy. I had to evolve and start fighting those hills in a smarter, more balanced way.*

Incline is one of the greatest tools a treadmill has to offer. It is also one of the most misused and misunderstood elements of treadmill training. Learn to do it right and you'll unlock the magic of a perfect run. Do it wrong, and the consequences range from frustrating to debilitating. You can seriously hurt yourself blasting too fast up a steep incline or doing too much incline work. There is the right incline for the right speed, and the method and workouts in this book prescribe it perfectly.

Let's be honest, hills suck! The inclines in our lives can range from annoying to downright impossible. After compiling a list of all the questions and concerns people had about incline and combining them with my own experience and research, I set out to find answers, real answers. The result of that work is perhaps the only comprehensive guide to incline treadmill running available, taking the "how to" to a whole new level. The incline principles of the BITE method are what I call the secret sauce, applying limits and modifications never seen before in a treadmill program. All of the runs formulated later in this book have a healthy dose of this secret sauce. Nothing is random, unbalanced, or uncalculated. The BITE method is designed to give you the perfect amount of incline to speed. That ratio is key—the right speed to the right incline. This guide pairs incline and speed to ensure you get the maximum benefits from incline training while reducing the overall stress on the body. It's a major win. As with the other BITE principles, I created an incline plan including numbers, scales, and running form that is concise and simple to understand and adopt but dramatic in its effect on the body. So many people sustain injuries while running inclines incorrectly, but when executed properly, they are an incomparable fat incinerator. With that in mind, I designed these principles to increase the benefits of incline running while decreasing the consequences.

## Impact of Incline—The Whole Story

In recent years there has been a rush of information supporting the benefits of adding incline to your treadmill run. The most popular of these benefits is the decrease in *impact* and *braking* forces acting on the body, which cause considerable wear and tear.

In the simplest terms, impact forces occur as you make initial contact with the treadmill. Braking forces take place just after that initial contact, as your body pushes into the ground. Both of these forces exist when you are running flat and increase dramatically on a decline. Braking forces are the harshest on your body. A study on these relationships called "Ground Reaction Forces During Downhill and Uphill Running" by Doctors Gottschall and Kram in 2005 showed running on a 9° decline caused a 73% increase in parallel braking forces. Essentially, too much downhill, too fast, will wreak havoc on your body, especially your knees. Luckily, there isn't a decline on a treadmill, and that wasn't a mistake.

*Incline reduces pressure on the knees.*

By contrast, these forces can be nearly eliminated when running on an incline. This is great news for you and your knees. You will notice a healthy dose of 1–5% inclines in the workouts in this book and in every BITE-inspired run. And like so many other treadmill workouts, I tremendously value the reduced impact on the body and increased muscle work that inclines induce. But *unlike* any other treadmill program, class, or workout, I'll let you in on a little secret—there is more to this story.

>>>

I remember the day I stood slumped on the treadmill after sprinting that impossibly steep incline. If incline is supposed to reduce impact, why did my body hurt so badly, even my knees? I took nearly every treadmill class I could find and realized two painfully obvious things: First, everyone assumed that if adding incline reduces impact, then more incline must be better. Reading factoids like this in magazines can mislead even expert runners and their instructors. Second, companies have become *so* obsessed with calorie-burn bragging rights that they are failing to understand running is an age-old art with a sophisticated science. It is not something from which information should be cherry-picked, abused, manipulated, or left for interpretation; attempts to do so will backfire, fueling the very fear of running they set out to eradicate in the first place.

I did not come up with a radical or hypothetical guideline to incline but rather a very practical one. After diving deep into running research I saw the same beneficial findings everyone else was seeing, but with the exception of one little red flag. There is another force acting on the body to consider when running—the *propulsive* force. Simply, this is the force that drives a runner forward. The average person can push off the ground with upward of 500 pounds of force, while a professional sprinter can push off with nearly 1,000 pounds of force. And unlike the other forces, it does not decrease with incline. On the contrary, the same study mentioned previously found a 75% increase in this force when running on an incline. And it was there I saw the missing part to the incline story. It makes perfect sense, as this is the force required at liftoff. Adding incline means you must now work against gravity, pushing upward as well as pushing forward.

>>>

While this undoubtedly contributes to a bigger calorie burn, nothing is without limits. The steeper the incline, the more compromised certain joints in your body will become, especially the ankles, hips, and lower back. For example, as the incline becomes steeper you will have to shorten the angle between your knee and your chest (excessively leaning forward), exposing your lower back to a less stable position. Your body has to do this in order to keep from falling backward, as the ground is no longer perpendicular to your body. You add to that more speed, which increases propulsive force, and you have created the perfect recipe for injury and a lifetime of aches and pains. You don't need to sprint on steep inclines to get the benefits of incline running. This is exactly why that sort of sprinting in the track-and-field world is reserved only for part of a conditioning phase during racing season. Racers are not sprint-training on steep inclines all the time. Based on this information, a closer look at which inclines produce the greatest propulsive force, and years of personal trial and observation, the BITE method gives you the most important incline guideline for treadmill training.

## The Right Incline for the Right Speed

Yes, it's that simple, and you won't hear it anywhere else. It is ultimately the most unique piece of information the BITE method offers to the world of treadmill running. Taking risk factors and effectiveness into account, top speeds for your ability are best reserved for inclines of 0–5%. This doesn't mean larger inclines aren't important, but rather they should be used with a signature and scientific formula of reduced speeds. You will mindfully learn to adjust speed and time to each incline in order to attain the best possible calorie burn with the least amount of stress on your body. You'll be amazed how much better you feel when you hit inclines with the proper speeds. Remember, the BITE method does not reduce the workload, but rather it spreads it out in a smoother, safer, and more maintainable way. The workouts in this book maintain this guideline strictly, and you will never be asked to sprint at your

*No maximum sprinting over a 5% incline.*

tops speeds on any inclines over 5%. Following are the optimal ranges of inclines and speeds that should be used for any treadmill workout:

- **0–5% incline—sprint speeds** (the top range of your maximum speeds)
- **6–8% incline—medium speeds** (difficult pace but not approaching max speeds)
- **9–12% incline—slow speeds** (considered easy, slow speeds)
- **12% incline and up** (use sparingly, and at very slow speeds/walks)

Because everyone has a different range of speed, you must assess your own ability and use your own perceived notion of what is slow, medium, and fast for you. The speed chapter coming up will describe how a slow, medium, and fast speed should feel. This is the responsible approach to using incline—telling you the whole story so that you can turn risk into amazing results.

## Importance of 0%

This is another element that the BITE method prescribes differently from many others. I do not believe that the reduction of braking forces justifies training on an incline all the time. We certainly don't live our lives that way, as we constantly need to walk down stairs, hills, and slopes. Earth is not flat—you go up, and you definitely go down. Your body is brilliant, and it will adapt to nearly any environment in which you put it. That being said, if you constantly train on an incline, you are going to lose strength in the stabilizing muscles needed the next time you are faced with any sort of decline. I see it all the time at the gym. We have all seen those people at the gym constantly maxing out incline, holding onto the treadmill for dear life, convinced they are saving their knees and getting a great workout. That addiction to incline so often leads to incline abuse, resulting in an inability to run flat or downhill without knee pain. Just as you are what you eat, you are how you run, and if you don't use your ability, you'll lose your ability.

*A 0% incline plays an important role.*

There are also a few myths floating around about incline. The biggest one is that the treadmill dips so far forward in the front that you *must* add incline to get the treadmill to be level. That idea is extremely outdated. Modern treadmills are not as front-heavy as their predecessors and are adjustable to make sure they are level, regardless of whether or not your floor is. Another defense people use is that adding a 1% incline will mimic the wind resistance found outdoors. First of all, if you want to feel like you are running outdoors, run outdoors. Second, for every head wind there is a tail wind that will make it easier when you turn around, essentially balancing out efforts and uprooting the resistance argument altogether. I tell people all the time, celebrate the differences between outdoor and indoor running rather than stressing over trying to make them the same.

## Balancing Incline

You don't need to understand how I blend incline into the workouts found in this book, but it is important for you to understand the science and logic on which it's based. After years of study I came up with an equation of balance for the principles of running so that when creating workouts, they have a foundation to grow from. Without it, there is nothing but randomness, guessing, and trial and error. Understanding the exchange between incline and speed allows us to make small changes outside of balance to create build and flow. It is the very first thing you will notice when you do the workouts in this book. They have an incredible flow that immediately engages your mind and progresses in a smooth and understandable way. I came up with a simple table that shows how speed should change to compensate for an increase or decrease in incline, creating great balance.

*A 1% change in incline is worth a +/−0.2 mph change in speed.*

The following table was used as a basis in creating the workouts in this book. Again, you don't need to understand this in-depth, but it will give you a better appreciation for the quality and sophistication of the workouts you'll be doing in this book.

| INTERVAL SPEED VS. INTERVAL INCLINE | | |
|---|---|---|
| 0.2 MPH SPEED CHANGE = +/−1% INCLINE CHANGE | | |
| Speed (mph) | Incline | Notes |
| Fastest (9 mph) | 0% | |
| −0.2 mph (8.8 mph) | 1% | |
| −0.2 mph (8.6 mph) | 2% | |
| −0.2 mph (8.4 mph) | 3% | |
| −0.2 mph (8.2 mph) | 4% | Fastest speeds okay below 5% |
| −0.2 mph (8 mph) | 5% | Medium speeds okay above 5% |
| −0.2 mph (7.8 mph) | 6% | |
| −0.2 mph (7.6 mph) | 7% | |
| −0.2 mph (7.4 mph) | 8% | |

If I go from a 2% incline to 1% incline in a workout and speed up a full 1 mph (instead of the recommended 0.2 mph increase in speed), I've made a jump so far outside of the balance from the previous table that I will have likely made the second interval far too difficult, or at the very least jarring. This table allows us to know when we are changing inclines at rates that are disproportionate to changes in speed. Thus, the incline foundation of the BITE method maintains that a 1% change in incline is worth a 0.2 mph change in speed. Sometimes the workouts in the book will evolve with perfect balance, but most often they will shift slightly outside of that balance to increase the amount of work and create new challenges, but all within reason. All incline workouts in this book were built precisely with these guidelines in mind so you will have the safest, smoothest run possible.

*Every time you raise the incline by 1% you must decrease your speed by 0.2 mph in order to do the same net work on each interval.*

Just like me you will never be 18 again, and just like me you'll never truly conquer a hill. You may get to the top or to the end of an incline interval, but you'll never beat it. While you become a stumbling, exhausted mess, the hill will remain completely unaffected by your efforts. But if we learn to respect the hill, we can begin to work with the hill instead of against it. With the tools in this chapter, and the runs throughout this book, you will transform your hate-hate relationship with inclines into a love-hate (the hate half never truly goes away). You will find a balanced way to quickly burn calories without compromising the overall well-being of your body. Gravity will always be a bitch. But if you attack an incline intelligently, purposefully, and respectfully, you will see great rewards.

## THE HILL REMAINS

*Just as I thought I would never have to see the Grand Valley State University ski hill again in my life, I did. Recently on a visit to GVSU, some 12 years after that last hill workout with my team, there I was again. The same head coach, Jerry Baltes, decided to take me for a "casual" run through campus, which is one of the most beautiful, inspiring campuses in the entire country. It was a lovely run, winding through trails and under tall oaks and maples. It was a very relaxing run until my coach led me through an opening in the trail and directly to the bottom of a hill. And there it was, that damn ski hill, exactly as I had left it 12 years ago. My coach grinned and we gave it a go. It was as horribly exhilarating as I remembered it.*

## KEY POINTS FROM CHAPTER 3

- Incline is important in taking pressure off the knees.

- No maximum sprinting on an incline over 5%.

- A 0% incline is a critical conditioning tool for overall health.

- The incline exchange says that a 1% change in incline is worth a +/−0.2 mph change in speed to create balanced work from interval to interval.

## Chapter 4

# SPEED—SMART IS THE NEW FAST

Throughout history, mankind has had an insatiable need for speed. Our obsession with high-speed Internet, flight time, zippy cars, and yes, our own bodies has created an endless quest to push boundaries and limits when it comes to speed. But unlike the Internet and a Boeing 757, you have the complexities of being organic. Getting faster is only a single facet of becoming a better runner and getting in better shape. The workouts in this book will make you a faster runner, but it's only when you begin to master all the other facets of running, such as endurance, recovery, and duration, that you truly unlock your greatest potential. I want this book to do more than help you reach that potential. I want it to remind you that once you do reach it, it is okay to celebrate it, to own it, to live in it for a very long time. The effectiveness of a treadmill workout is not determined by how much harder you can make it, which too often is the goal of treadmill workouts, but rather how often you are able to do it. Sustainability in running is the key to improvement, to a better body, and to getting faster.

# THE FINAL RACE

*On May 23, 2003, I found myself walking to the starting line of what would become the race that taught me the boundaries of potential. It was also the final race of my college racing career. It was an emotional and life-changing moment. My race consisted of only two very fast, very physical laps around the track. It was the NCAA National Championships at Southern Illinois University Edwardsville. I was a senior and the only male runner representing my team that year, so the pressure, as well as the hot Illinois sun, was heavy. It all happened so fast. I remember the gun going off, and then I remember suddenly approaching the final turn. It was the last race of my college career, and I could hear my coach yelling, "Now David! You have to go now!" I had never raced against such talent. But I had just come off a school record and my ego was flying sky-high. Still, time was running out. My coach was right. I had to move up, even though I had possibly already waited too long. It was time to use the speed I had been saving. I squeezed my fists, let out a strange animal-like sound, and put 4 years of hard training on the line. I had sacrificed so much for this one moment. My heart, consumed by adrenaline, thrashed against my chest. This was it, I told myself, and I lowered my chin and began making the final move of my college career. I was going to qualify for the finals. Then, suddenly, something was wrong, terribly wrong. . . .*

It is an undeniable truth that we will eventually slow down, have a bad day, or at the very least reach our fastest potential. The speed of your youth that you thought would always last will eventually fade. If it hasn't, I assure you, it someday will. And although I cannot stop time, or promise you will win a race, I have discovered a way to rethink speed so that you can still feel the rush, without the loss. It's time that we have an honest conversation about speed. There is no running program or method in the world that can promise you will continue to get faster indefinitely. It will not happen. So let's put aside false promises and misleading pitches and get to work on you being the fastest, most kick-ass runner you can be. Using the tools in this book you will unlock your greatest potential, with workouts specifically designed to help you find your best speed. I assure you, you will be faster than you were before you did the workouts in this book. But more importantly, you will learn how to run smarter, so that when you realize you aren't the carefree 18-year-old you once were, you will have a few tricks up your sleeve to keep you lean, healthy, and running for a lifetime.

## Speed Cushion

Speed cushioning is probably the best tool I have created to help you balance speed. The idea is simple: Bring down your fastest speed just a bit, and balance that with a slightly faster recovery, essentially creating less of a gap between your top and bottom speeds. Say you are able to hit a maximum speed of 10 mph for 1 minute and then recover for 1 minute at 4 mph. Often this "pedal to the metal" speed work leaves people feeling terrible the next day, full of aches and pains. The idea of cushioning is to slow down your maximum speed up to a full point and bring up your recovery between 1–2 full points. So, you would try a sprint of 9 mph (–1 mph from last sprint) and a recovery of 5.5 mph (+1.5 mph from last recovery).

*Decrease your fast speed slightly and increase recovery speed.*

| Interval | Interval Speed | Recovery Speed |
|---|---|---|
| 1 minute | 10 mph | 4 mph |
| 1 minute with cushioning | 9 mph (−1 mph) | 5.5 mph (+1.5 mph) |

Modesty aside, years of training have given me the ability to sprint at maximum 12+ mph, and although I can, I choose not to. I choose to bring down my maximum to 11–11.5 mph and bring up my recovery to 5–8 mph. This allows me to keep the same great burn but feels so much better on my body, during the workout and after.

You won't do less work; you'll simply spread the workload out in a smoother, more effective way. It is still a form of intense interval training, toasting the same calories, just in a safer, less painful, and more sustainable method for treadmill training. In addition, this is the reality in the competitive world of running. Those lean, mean running machines you see on TV did not get there by just sprinting all out and walking during practice. They got there by also doing intervals at percentages of their top race speed (pace), and pairing them with challenging, meaningful, and calculated recoveries. If this creates some of the fastest human beings in the world, with bodies any of us would want, we can surely adopt the concept of active recoveries for our treadmill training. Cushioning is really just the simplified version of maintaining some work during the recoveries. You'll still feed your need for speed and you will recover, but not to the extremes of both ends. The result is a more balanced approach to speed, again maintaining your burn, bringing down the impact and stress associated with constant sprint work, and feeling better when the sun rises the next day. And remember, running is like many things in life: It isn't always the fastest car that gets there first; it's the one that took the smarter route.

## Starting Speed

Your Personal Best is simply the fastest you can safely go for 1 minute. Basically it's your max, the speed that you can't maintain for longer than 1 minute without stepping off. Choosing the right starting speed is one of the most important things to master when treadmill training. You get that part right, and any treadmill workout can be transformed into an entirely new experience. I developed and have been using this pacing method for almost a decade now, and this placement of speed and using appropriate numbers for your specific circumstances makes this method work for everyone. Once you understand the right speed range for your ability, you will be able to simply plug your speeds into any of the preprogrammed workouts in Part Two of this book. The single best way to find your starting speed is to learn what your top limits are. The BITE method calls this your Personal Best (PB). After trying just one run, you'll quickly discover your current PB, giving you a reference for every workout in this book. It takes the stress out of knowing if you are

*Your starting speed is strictly dependent on your Personal Best.*

starting too fast or too slow. All the workouts are programmed to grow and change based on that PB, so you can trust the workout is balanced and focus on arriving at the final destination in each workout. In no time your PB will advance, and you will discover potential you never knew you had. While there is no perfect calculation to find that PB, this chapter will present a reference table, giving you the recommended PB ranges based on experience. Everyone falls into one of these categories, and after just one workout, you'll know exactly where you fall on the speed spectrum. Learning *your* exact ability is the only honest way to learn pacing and start interval training like a pro.

Most programs categorize you as a beginner, intermediate, or advanced runner. I have been desperately trying to change that conversation. It's just not right. I have this client I work with on a treadmill. He is 75 years old with a hip replacement and in many programs his top speeds fall into a traditional "beginner" category. He told me one day that the only reason he comes to my class is because I was the first person who didn't call him a beginner or treat him like a 5-year-old just because he isn't fast anymore. It was an emotional and powerful moment that set the stage for a healthier conversation. You see, for me and this method, there are no beginners, and I'll be damned if I'm ever going to look a 75-year-old in the eyes and call him one! He has been through more in his life than I could ever imagine. It's time that someone also showed you, regardless of your ability, the respect and dignity you deserve. And even if you're someone who doesn't care about being called a beginner or intermediate or even advanced, let me assure you, learning your personal speed range is still much better than learning a category someone else throws you into. You will see results faster than any other way, guaranteed. It is the only way to be empowered to take back control of your own workout.

That being said, I do understand that categorizing can make my job easier—hell, that's why most treadmill coaches do it, not to be mean to you but to make it easy for them. And I'm certain you would love to just be told what speed to start at. The less thinking you have to do the better, right? Wrong! While that may work in other facets of your health-and-fitness life, running is different. You must learn how to pace yourself based on *your* ability, not a group or demographic that you get thrown into. Once you take control of your own starting speed and your own destination, thinking will turn to engagement, and that is the healthiest thing you could ever do on a treadmill: be engaged in your workout. After speaking with mental health experts, I feel confident that this engagement is one of the major contributing factors in the impressive new findings of Alzheimer's and dementia risk reduction in those who run. You won't ever realize it, but your mind must process huge amounts of information and make hundreds of calculations and decisions in order to acclimate to changes in speed and incline. This is a very healthy exercise for your brain. To enhance this benefit, I intentionally created workouts that have a network of disguised mathematical patterns and connections that require you to think about what speed to set rather than being told. Although I am certainly no Mozart, this is very much what he did. Many mathematicians believe the hidden mathematical connections and relationships found in his music lead to "mental enhancement for the listener." A well-orchestrated run can do the same thing for you, enhancing your mood and keeping your mind sharp through engagement. Now if I could only get you to listen to Mozart *while* doing the BITE workouts in this book, your gray matter would be as fit as your abs!

You will be the person in control, and only when that happens will you be able to start doing wicked smart work that will change your body faster than you ever thought possible. Finding your speed range isn't as hard as you might think. Nearly every person falls within the following "top speed" ranges. For the first run in the Three-Week Kick-Start, you will estimate your speed range based on your experience. Assess how you feel at the end of the run. It's alarming how quickly a person will say, I know exactly how much faster I could have gone, or how much slower I should have gone. It's an important moment of discovery. And if you really want the ultimate treadmill workout, this is how you find it. Remember, this is just a guide to get you started. I promise, after just one workout, you will know so much about your ability and what top speed range you fall into. Every workout in this book is designed and created backward based exactly on your own Personal Best ending speed. That is not only empowering, but it is also critical to utilizing pacing in any great treadmill workout. Learning to pace yourself, especially on a treadmill, is the real game-changer!

- **4–6 mph for 1 minute**—PB for those who consider themselves new to running or with physical limitations
- **6–8 mph for 1 minute**—PB for those who consider themselves novice to occasional runners
- **8–10 mph for 1 minute**—PB for those who consider themselves experienced and frequent runners
- **10 mph and up for 1 minute**—PB for those at a high level of conditioning and experience

## Tips on Speed

It is important to know when you are running too fast. Besides being discouraging, it can be extremely dangerous. Two things happen if you are going too fast. One, you step off the treadmill early because you consistently can't finish the interval. Or, your form starts to degrade to an unsafe point where you start sitting back on your hips and you feel like you are reaching forward to hold on. If you feel out of control, you are going too fast, and running out of control is not worth it. There is a fine line between pushing yourself through exhaustion and pushing yourself to a breaking point.

*Out of control is not good speed work.*

### Top Speed

Sprinting at top speeds should always be reserved for the last half of your workout. The systematic and gradual build of speed is the safest and healthiest way to achieve top speeds. This contributes to TreadFlow and is extremely fun and addictive, training the mind to be sharp and disciplined as well. The workouts in this book never begin with a sprint, ever. In most runs, you will actually only hit your stop speed one time at the finish line of your workout. It's all the work you did before that that is most meaningful.

### Adjusting Speed

The great thing about using this form of pacing is that it is easy to adjust. Once you learn your Personal Best speed it is easy to manipulate if you are having a rough week, or you feel ready to challenge yourself to hit a new PB. The workouts I have created in the book are set up for you to succeed and conquer, and you will only rarely have to adjust your speed range. If you ever do feel like you need to, I always recommend shifting down or up your PB reference 0.5 mph depending on how you are feeling, and then continuing with the workout with that adjustment. Making too big of an adjustment is most often regrettable.

## THE FINISH LINE

*Years ago, on a hot day in Illinois, I learned one of the most valuable lessons I've ever learned about speed. There was nothing wrong with me physically, but rather I had misjudged my competition. As in my previous races, I thought I could save all my speed for the end, for the final kick. That's where things went terribly wrong—as I made that final turn shifting into fifth gear to pass my competition. The problem was, some of the other guys had a sixth gear that I didn't see coming. On top of that, I was simply out of gas that day. No matter how hard I tried, the world around me turned to quicksand. The panic set in that this was how I would finish my running career. I kept trying to surge forward, but one step at a time, I watched the race slip through my hands. I had never felt so heavy in my life. I could hardly lift my feet off the ground in the final 100 meters. I could not catch the guys in front of me. As I crossed the final finish line of my track career, I looked over at my less-than-happy coach and I knew he had been right. That was another valuable lesson in life: When you have great coaches, you need to trust and listen to them! I didn't have the speed to "save it for the end." If I had just used my speed a bit earlier, it may have been an entirely different outcome. I had to run that race differently, and my ego got in the way. I fell to my knees, feeling the sting of the sun-baked track, and let the smell of burnt rubber fill my nose. I stumbled off the track, got an understanding hug from our middle-distance coach, Jill Stamison, and then sobbed alone, with the reality that I had gone as fast as I was likely ever meant to go. A close friend of mine, a standout Division*

*1 basketball player, reminded me once that an athlete dies twice in his life; once when he actually dies, and once when he plays that final game. It is so painfully true.*

While most of us are not professional sprinters, we still deserve to feel the freedom and exhilaration of running at our best. While it's important to have a hunger to be better, to be faster, it is also okay to know your limits. There will be a race or a treadmill run one day when you simply can't go any faster. That's life, and it's completely okay. So, instead of breaking yourself by pursuing that constant need for more speed, open up to the opportunity of sprinting smarter, not faster. Once you're able to do that, you'll stop stressing about how fast you used to be, and start celebrating how fast you can be now. There are many ways to win a race; don't forget that.

## KEY POINTS FROM CHAPTER 4

- Cushioning is bringing down your fastest speed slightly and increasing recovery speed. A more challenging recovery is often a healthier and more effective choice than seeking more speed.

- Learn pacing by calculating your starting speed based on strictly knowing how the run ends and on your Personal Best.

## Chapter 5

# *DURATION—TOO SHORT VS. TOO LONG*

How long can you run? Treadmill workouts prescribe nearly every range of intervals, from 10-second sprints, to 5-minute hills. The ranges are as varied as the reasons you are getting on a treadmill, be it training for a long-distance race, trying to become a better sprinter, or because it's a blizzard outside. I knew, however, there had to be a "best" range for someone using the treadmill to burn fat and get faster. When I was training for the 800-meter sprint, I remember how specific the training intervals were to our group of half-milers. In order to achieve the results we needed to succeed in our event, our coach had created a very effective range of interval workouts that gave us our best chance at success. After years of observing different programs, looking at how certain intervals change the body, both physically and mentally, I created an interval range that is optimal for any treadmill workout. Getting your timing right is so critical for achieving results.

# AGAINST THE CLOCK

*On May 3, 2003, a few weeks before my disastrous NCAA race, I had my last qualifying race at Saginaw Valley State University. You see, in college track, you don't qualify for the national championships as a team; you must qualify as an individual. It can be an immense amount of pressure for any college athlete. I had never been more nervous in my entire life. I had not yet qualified and so I toed the line for what was a final chance to qualify for nationals. If I did not run fast enough it would all be over. I was scared to death for my college running career to be over. I loved racing and being with my team more than just about anything in my life. Consumed by nerves and fear, I trembled as the gun went off. We were off, quick but controlled, and I quickly settled into third position. I had a plan; I knew my competition. Four years of intense, specific training, 4 years of building a war chest of endurance. It was going to work. It had to.*

*One lap down and my endurance was proving effective; I had not lost a single stride or a second off my pace. And then it was time. I surged with everything I had in my legs and in my heart. I quickly passed the guy in front of me, but it was not important. I had to run the last 200 meters in under 28 seconds or it was completely over. Every mile I had ever run, every drop of sweat had come down to this—it was me against the clock. I barreled down the final homestretch, driving and fighting to hold on to the only life I knew.*

It is all about the clock. You can make incline and speed go away, but time is the one unavoidable variable of running and life. It doesn't stop for anyone. To utilize the principles of speed, incline, and recovery you must understand the timing of all these variables. In addition, it is the often the clever and surprising "timing" elements in the BITE method that turn casual runners into addicts. This healthy obsession with timing creates smart, dedicated, goal-oriented running. The BITE method applies some very simple but very specific and effective guidelines on duration to guarantee your timing is perfect.

## The Perfect Interval

Years of studying the benefits of certain interval lengths have led to this simple guideline for any treadmill workout. These intervals have proven to be extraordinarily effective yet sustainable when used on a treadmill. The BITE method prescribes this interval time frame as the most effective use of your time. For most people, anything under 30 seconds needs to be relatively aggressive to require work, and anything over 2 minutes can create emotional stress and often becomes quite boring as well. Save the super-short sprints for the track and save the long runs for the trail. Every workout in this book follows this important guideline.

*All intervals should fall between 30 seconds and 2 minutes.*

## Lead Time

The biggest mistake people make when using a treadmill is they start late by waiting for the machine to rev up. And it breaks my heart to see other coaches let this slide. All treadmills must speed up to the set speed, and that can take anywhere from 5 to 15 seconds, depending on how fast you are asking the treadmill to go. I see it everywhere—someone starts the clock on a 30-second sprint then speeds up, but actually ends up doing less than 15 seconds of the actual work they were trying to achieve. To solve this problem, simply always start speeding up about 10 seconds before every interval. You may feel like you are eating a little into your recovery time, but that will make you much stronger and more fit than eating into your interval time.

*Speed up about 10 seconds before every interval.*

## Recovery Time

We will discuss this more in the recovery chapter, but it is really important to understand that to get the most out of your time and to use the proven method in this book, you must be just as diligent about timing your recovery as you were with your interval. Random, loose recoveries do not exist in the great running programs of the world, and they shouldn't exist in your treadmill program either. The pros don't check e-mails between intervals and neither should you. Although the majority of recoveries are 1 minute, they do sometimes change to become shorter and longer to complement the work done on the interval. It can be challenging at first to keep track of intermittent 45-second recovery times, for example, but taking the time to get good at it is worth the effort and will set your workouts apart from everyone else's. The recovery time is calculated to be part of the workout, so if you "chill" on a recovery here and there you are breaking the balance of work and will slow down your progress. Besides, staying closely engaged with your clock is what makes the workout go by so fast—you don't have time for distractions or boredom.

*Recovery durations are not flexible— they are as exact as the interval.*

## TIME DOESN'T STOP

*The clock doesn't wait for anyone; it is the inevitable truth of life. That qualifying race in May of 2003 was that truth for me. I had 200 meters to go and an exact pace I had to keep if I had any hope of making it to nationals. The cheering and screaming from my teammates filled my heart and carried me across the finish line. I had calculated the exact time and duration I had to run. I looked over to the timing station and saw a grin on my coach's face. "You did it, Siik. You're going to nationals . . . and by the way, that was also a school record." My heart leapt from my chest. I ran smart, I respected the clock, and it paid off big. I want that for you as well! So now it's time for you to start making every second on that treadmill mean something, so that you cross the finish line with victory and a little extra time for the other things in your life!*

## KEY POINTS FROM CHAPTER 5

- All intervals should fall between 30 seconds and 2 minutes.

- Speed up about 10 seconds before every interval.

- Recovery durations are not flexible—they are as exact as the interval.

## Chapter 6

# RECOVERY— NOT ALWAYS EASY

Making your recovery periods more meaningful is one of the greatest lessons you could ever learn in running. It is also one of the biggest secrets to success on the treadmill. Far too many treadmill programs focus on putting all the work on the interval and leaving the recovery period up to you. While this may be an exciting and popular method in other areas of fitness, it is a big mistake in running. You see, in the world of running the recovery period is still part of your workout. You don't check out, take a seat, or walk around as slowly as you want. There seems to be this misunderstanding that *recovery* means, "complete recovery." Although there are purposeful times when that may be true, rarely is that the goal. Focusing on making your recovery more challenging instead of maxing out the treadmill every time on the interval is not only a massive calorie burn but will help you build an endurance so great, it will affect nearly every aspect of your life. The strongest, fittest runners in the world take smart, calculated, and precise recovery periods when they work out. Almost half your time is spent recovering in a treadmill workout, so it is wise to make it meaningful.

## ACTIVE RECOVERY IS SMART RECOVERY

*It was a slushy and cold January day on the streets of New York, but I was sweating buckets on a dimly lit treadmill. Music blasted through the speakers, and a very fit and motivating instructor yelled out instructions. It was a hard run, but I had the convenience of knowing exactly how to keep any run under control. However, I did feel a little bad for those around me who seemed under the spell that the more extreme the interval, the better.*

*We had just started the second to last interval, and I was laser-focused. Then suddenly, as if the music had stopped and there were a spotlight over my head, I heard my name being called out on the speakers. I get a little used to being picked on, usually all in good fun. Since I'm a treadmill geek, everyone loves an opportunity to examine my every move. The instructor's words soared across the room, and I realized all eyes were on me. "Come on David Siik, is that all you've got? I thought you were this big treadmill runner. The guys on both sides of you are running faster than you." I smiled at the instructor, but I did not change my speed. Then, in the final seconds of the interval the guys beside me began adding as much speed as they could, misunderstanding, perhaps, the instructor's intentions. With painfully bad form they both looked over at my monitor to see if I was going to match their speeds. They wanted a race for sure, but little did they know I had already won the race, many intervals ago. The instructor screamed the countdown, 10 . . . 9 . . . 8 . . . and, as expected, the guy on my left jumped off onto the sides of the treadmill, the belt still howling between his legs. Shortly after followed the guy on my right. This jumping ship early is simply quitting early, usually because you are going way too fast or you have decided doing part of the interval is good enough. Could you imagine if Usain Bolt decided to stop just a few meters before the finish line? Of course not, and I don't want it to happen to you. Usually we step off to the sides early on a treadmill because our mind gives out and tells us to quit. To fix this you need to either bring down your speed to one that you can actually accomplish for the entire interval time or work on your mental endurance. With the workouts in this book, I hope to show you how to do both. As I brought my speed down (after the interval was actually over) to a very challenging but functional recovery speed, the guys clapped and cheered for each other, continuing to stand on the sides of the treadmill, undoubtedly excited to tweet about how fast they had just run for 1 minute (or 51 seconds, according to the clock). They eventually started walking, wincing at my monitor as if I didn't hear we were supposed to be recovering. I heard all right, and I was recovering, but I was making that recovery mean something.*

Recovery is perhaps the most misunderstood and underappreciated principle of treadmill running. It is the BITE method's attention to recovery that sets it apart from any other program. All successful outdoor-running programs have recoveries that are meaningful, with intention and purpose. Treadmill running should not be different. The BITE method of running brings down the often reckless intensities of the intervals and shifts the placement of work a little more onto the recoveries. This is the "cushioning" concept introduced to you in Chapter 4. This idea creates a comparable net workload and calorie burn but with a more gradual and balanced placement of that work. You get stronger faster and without the pain in your knees, hips, and back. It may sound difficult to find how much recovery is the right amount to keep your burn going, but really it is something you will learn quickly with the BITE guidelines to help you.

*Your first recovery must be a minimum of 50% of your first interval speed.*

## The 50% Recovery Rule

After your first interval, you should be able to maintain a minimum of 50% of your fast speed for a recovery speed. This rule applies to only the first segment of a workout (as you'll need more recovery later) and is simply based on only the speed you do for your first interval. For example, if your starting interval speed was 8 mph, the slowest your recovery speed should be is 4 mph. If you can't maintain at least 4 mph, you are going too fast and you will likely not be able to safely finish the workout as designed. It's that simple. Choose a slightly slower fast speed until you can maintain half of it on a recovery. I created this rule largely for the runners I found myself running next to on that cold slushy day in New York City. It really helps keep things under control, reduces the likeliness of injury, and is actually more work, which produces more results! Remember, just because your car can go 120 mph doesn't mean that's how fast you should take it around every corner.

Many with sprinting speeds below 7 mph will find this rule easy to follow and will likely recover at a much faster pace than 50% of their first interval speed. And that is great! It doesn't mean you have to recover at exactly 50% of your first interval speed, just that you shouldn't go below it. If your fast speed is 5 mph, for example, pairing it with a 2.5 mph recovery will likely feel too slow. I encourage you to choose a more challenging recovery speed whenever it feels right for you.

## The Perfect Recovery

The right recovery is the one that allows you to feel back in control just in time for the next interval. Many of the workouts in this book have dynamic recoveries, changing in incline, duration, and even speed to maintain the added element of a "working" recovery. If the workout doesn't give you an exact speed for the recovery time, or you're in a treadmill class and the instructor just says "recover," you need to find the speed that allows you to get your breathing back under control but doesn't allow you to rest more than you need to. Remember, this method is the sweet spot between sprint training and distance training, and the recovery should be between them as well. I always recommend that people attempt to commit to a recovery that feels slightly uncomfortable

*Take what you need to recover, and only what you need.*

but is enough to allow them to succeed in the next interval. If the intervals get too challenging toward the end of the run, and you feel you can no longer maintain the recovery speed you have been holding, try taking it down 0.5 mph at a time as needed. Remember, the 50% recovery rule applies only to the first segment of any workout in this book. You *will* need more recovery as a workout progresses, and herein lies the balance of recovery. Learning to take only what you need in a recovery can completely transform how you feel after the run, and the increase in overall intensity and calorie burn during the workout will shock you.

## Post-Run Recovery

Running can be a lot of work, which is largely why the less motivated opt for other workouts. Running really is a full-body workout in which you must take proper rest periods. This is the recovery you take after and between the workouts. I always recommend you do not do more than 2 days of treadmill intervals in a row. It doesn't mean you have to completely take a day off from working out. Rather, do a lower-impact workout such as weight training, yoga, or cycling after multiple days of intervals. I am also a firm believer that you still must find at least one day of complete rest to let your body repair and strengthen. A complete rest day is a great day to stretch and restore your body. Personally, because I know I won't be working out on my rest days, I choose those days to reflect on my diet and make sure I'm eating right.

*For a runner, rest is critical to success.*

Changing how you recover can revolutionize the way you run, and it will remind you that it is often what you do when no one is looking that wins the race. I remember that cold, slushy day that I got picked on for letting the guys next to me run faster. I also remember getting ready to go into the final interval. While the tweeting runners to my left and right walked at a snail's pace, laughing and talking away, I was silent, stealthy, and in it to win it. I maintained the challenging recovery speed and prepared to roll into the next and final interval. The instructor bellowed across the room, "This is your last one. Go for it!" Of course, the guys next to me started late and stepped off early, but they made sure at some point to max out the speed of the treadmill, because in their eyes bragging rights over their speeds were the most valuable outcome of the workout. The well-meaning instructor did not celebrate my speed, or give me a shout-out or a pat on the back, although my interval speed was only 0.5 under the other runners' max. I didn't receive an award for starting each interval on time and not quitting early. There was no mention of my impressive ability to recover. And that's okay, because knowing you won is a hell of a lot better than needing someone to tell you that you did. The instructor walked the length of the treadmills calling out and celebrating mileage results and pace averages. As he got to me and my two Twitter friends he froze in front of my treadmill. The other guys shook their heads as if I had cheated. I ran infinitely more mileage, burned more calories, and had the stamina, the healthy heart and lungs, and frankly, the six-pack to prove it. So, let someone else tweet about how fast they are; you just worry about running smart, and in the long run, you will always win. Oh, and for the record, I tweeted after the workout as well, but mine said, "Poor guy next to me #StartedLate #SteppedOffEarly and still #ThinksHeWon!"

## KEY POINTS FROM CHAPTER 6

- Active recovery is smart recovery.

- Your first recovery must be a minimum of 50% of your first interval speed.

- Take what you need, and only what you need.

- Follow the recovery times that are given exactly.

## Chapter 7

# FORM—CRITICAL MISTAKES ON THE TREADMILL

Good running form is everything. It will revolutionize your experience on the treadmill and literally change the way your body looks. It will also decrease the chance of embarrassing yourself in the gym. In this chapter I will not only guide you toward better running form, but I will also explain to you *why* it makes a difference. There are likely many treadmill-specific mistakes you never knew you were making, and I will help you correct them.

## ONLY FOOLS RUSH IN

*There was this one treadmill that I loved running on in New York. It wasn't the best treadmill in the world, but I loved it because it had mirrors in the front and on one side but still had one side open to the rest of the gym. One part of my ego loved being able to see my strong running form in the mirrors, and the other loved that people in the gym could see how fast I was. I was newer to running on the treadmill, but coming off my college racing I was still fast and strong. I was just so pleased with myself. And then one day, I was served some humble pie.*

*I remember three things from that wicked cold day in New York. I remember someone I had a crush on walking past my treadmill and of course I sped up as fast as the treadmill would go, a complete act of machismo. I also remember seeing myself in the mirror and thinking how strong and powerful my stride looked. I was so ridiculously in love with myself. And then, I remember hearing a thump, the belt letting out the loudest screech I'd ever heard, and then—the stumble. As if I'd stepped out of a speeding car, my body cartwheeled into a knot, flying off the back of the treadmill, smashing into the wall behind me, and knocking the wind out of my chest so hard I thought I'd never breathe again. Cupping my skinned knee I looked up as I heard people trying desperately not to laugh. "Are you okay?" concerned voices asked from all around. And by simply running too close to the front of my treadmill and tripping on the front piece of plastic, I had lost all hope of ever asking that person out on a date.*

*I was officially the guy at the gym who fell on his ass. . . .*

## Proper Form

Everyone does it. There is a comfort and feeling of safety when you hug the front of your treadmill, belly pressed tight against the monitor. The problem is, you are literally running into a wall. You may not realize it, but running that close up causes major problems with your form. Most importantly, it limits your range of motion, preventing you from ever running with your natural stride and arm drive. You will have a tendency to swing your arms in a short, choppy motion. This causes a chain reaction down your body, resulting in a great amount of tension in the back, shoulders, and neck.

*Don't run too close to the front of your treadmill.*

All you need to do, especially on your sprints, is move back a few inches from the front of your treadmill. You should always try to sprint in the middle of your treadmill, allowing your body to run free without limitations. Try it sometime. Run fast really close to the front of the treadmill and then just allow yourself to creep back a bit on the treadmill. You will be shocked by how different it feels, and more importantly how much better it feels. Also, even though it is rare, some people find being on a moving treadmill can make them feel dizzy or unstable. Usually that problem goes away after just a couple of workouts as your body acclimates to the feeling of moving while the ground does not. You can also fix a lot of this with good form. Make sure you are not looking down at the belt. It strains your neck and can cause you to feel dizzy. Make sure to look out at the upper part of your treadmill and not around the room in a daydream. Again, most unsteady feelings take care of themselves as your body quickly adapts to this new environment of running.

### Foot Strike

There are many coaching philosophies on foot strike. There are entire books written on it, as well as clinics and certifications on method and form. This book is not designed to convince you one method is better than another. Instead, I will share with you my method of balance, based on natural movement and anatomy of the body, which has helped keep me running strong and injury-free my entire running career.

Contrary to some running methods that propose you always run on your forefoot (the front part of your foot), I believe, based on natural design, there is a balance of when you should forefoot strike and when you should heel strike. You are born with a fat pad on your heel called the calcaneal fat pad, which has the sole purpose (pun intended) of acting as a cushioning pad for your heel. Human beings, by natural design, will strike with this fat pad first when they are walking, jogging, or running at moderate speeds. When your heel touches down your body weight rolls toward the outside of your foot, where you also have a fat pad. From there your body weight moves to the forefoot fat pad, which is where you will push off the ground to take your next step. Look at the bottom of your foot and you'll see the perfect design and pattern of cushion that is built for this "heel-to-toe" foot strike.

Studies, like the one from the journal *Medicine and Science in Sports and Exercise* conducted in 2014 titled "Relationship Between Running Speed and Initial Foot Contact Patterns," have shown that as some runners accelerate, their foot strikes naturally move farther up the foot onto the forefoot. This natural adjustment is genius. For one, only striking with the front part of your foot means less contact with the ground, which means less friction, which is a positive when building speed. Second, speed increases force, and by landing on the forefoot you will engage shock-absorbing muscles of the lower limbs such as the calves and soleus. Striking with your heel when sprinting can essentially radiate more shock upward to the knee, whereas landing farther up on the forefoot allows your lower limb muscles and tendons to absorb a great deal of that shock.

So, in summary, at slower speeds it is acceptable to have the natural and instinctive "heel-to-toe" roll of rear foot striking. As you start to accelerate, it is best to land farther up onto your forefoot, for both efficiency and reduced shock and impact on the knees.

### Stride

This is another hot topic. There are a few things that all running coaches can agree on, and I do want to talk about that. Overstriding is bad for you. I am guilty of doing this on occasion. Overstriding is when you start reaching your legs in front of you to excessively lengthen your stride. The problem with this is that your foot is landing in front of your body weight as opposed to underneath you. It's like doing a lunge with bad form. Overstriding can be hard on your knees and hips. I do see it happen on the treadmill more often than on the street. I attribute this to the fact that the treadmill is creating a moving ground underneath you and your mind is calculating its stride for the pace you are trying to go. This causes some people to overcompensate for the moving treadmill. It also happens when runners get excited or are attempting to power through fatigue. Just make sure that your feet are landing as close to underneath you as possible.

On the flip side, many coaches have adopted a strategy of increased cadence, which basically equates to shortening your stride and taking more steps per minute. I absolutely agree that biomechanically this shorter stride can reduce force and impact on the body. It makes complete sense. I don't, however, believe in overcoaching and forcing cadence changes. First of all, it isn't natural. If a bear were chasing you, you would likely increase your stride length to accelerate. For most of us, the act of increasing our repetition and shortening our stride to reach that same speed is not a natural thing, which is why a coach has to teach a runner how to do it. I also have concerns that if you are always using an increased cadence you are never fully releasing the energy in your hip flexor region, which has a healthy and natural range of motion. Your gait and your stride are unique to you; no one ever has to teach you what they are. For this reason, I believe in a balance. I support taking slightly smaller strides at times to be a little kinder on your knees, but I also believe when sprinting, a full natural stride is important, beneficial, and, for many runners like me, efficient and pain-free.

The only time I want to be sure you do not run with a long, full stride is on hills. Studies have shown the human body gradually takes smaller and smaller strides as inclines get higher and higher. This smaller stride helps protect the knees, hips, and lower back. You should naturally be shortening your stride on steep hills, but in case you have ever been misinformed, you do *not* ever stride out on a steep incline. It requires a great amount of force to run steep inclines, and you want to be certain you are taking small, short, protective strides as you tackle the hill.

### Posture

Because of the repetitive nature of running, posture is important. One small bad habit can turn into a large problem when you are doing it mile after mile. Fortunately the treadmill creates the perfect environment to assess your posture and fix any of those other bad habits.

Running coaches often talk about tilt, or forward "lean." It is important to make sure that your torso weight is shifted ever so slightly over and in front of the hips, as opposed to behind. Think of it this way: You want to push your body weight instead of pull your body weight. When you are tilting ever so slightly forward while running you are engaging the strong muscles of the back and core to stabilize your body and help absorb shock. Remember that your muscles don't act only to produce power; they also absorb an incredible amount of energy to reduce shock and impact as you move. If you are sitting back on your hips, which usually happens as a result of fatigue, you are not engaging those important muscles of the back and you are letting your spine take on more impact than it needs to. This can lead to spinal compression and a slew of other back pains. Here is the best way to understand this: Stand up tall with your legs shoulder-width apart and place your palms on your lower back above your hips. Rest back on your hips and feel the soft, relaxed nature of the muscles on each side of the spine. Then, with your hands still on your back, tilt slightly forward with your chest. You will immediately feel the muscles that protect the spine engage (the erector spinae). Do this a couple of times to feel the difference, sitting back and relaxed, then tilting forward and feeling those muscles flex hard like a rock. You want those muscles working when you are running to help stabilize your upper torso and absorb shock away from the spine. Be careful not to overlean, however, as leaning too far forward can actually strain those muscles. The previous exercise shows you that you have to "tilt" only slightly forward to get those muscles onboard.

The other mistake people make on a treadmill is they look up and over their treadmill trying to watch TV. If this is you, stop! Treadmill manufacturers are no dummies, and they place the monitors in the best neutral position for varying heights so that you aren't straining your neck. Sounds like no big deal, but tilting your head back too much can be the primary culprit of a stiff and achy neck. Remember that you are designed to look out and slightly down to see the terrain in front of you. The place to keep your eye line is usually at the top of your monitor, which will keep your head in just the right position.

### Arms

This is one of my favorite topics. Fixing your arm drive can really change your run. Intense interval training is a killer workout for your arms. If you're a woman looking for long, lean arms or a guy looking for that ripped back and shoulders, using your arms during a run can help define the upper-body muscles.

The biggest mistake people make is that they swing their arms left to right across their centerline. It's easier that way, taking less energy and less effort. The problem with that is you're missing the opportunity for a great full-body workout and you could be creating future health problems. Excessive side-to-side arm swinging causes a twisting and pivoting motion in the hips, which over time can cause tightness, pain, and serious issues with the hips and lower back.

Here is the science. Your body is magnificent, and you were designed to have an opposite arm to complement the opposite leg. This is the reason human beings walk, jog, and run with an opposite-arm, opposite-leg movement instead of same-arm, same-leg. You see, when you drive your right leg upward in a sprint you create an immense amount of torque. Torque is a twisting force that is generated in your body when you lift one leg at a time. This torque causes your body to want to twist near your midsection when walking and running. If you suddenly did not have your left arm available to counterbalance that force from the right leg, you would likely lift off the ground, spin counter-clockwise, and fall flat on your face. Your opposite arm swings to counterbalance the force created from the opposite leg. This is the counterbalancing action that helps deal with torque, keeping you from dangerously twisting your hips. Here is a simple exercise that shows this. Run in place with high knees (creating force with your legs) while you lock your arms straight down at your sides, preventing them from swinging. You will immediately feel your upper body struggling and twisting from side to side. Then, keep up the high knees but slowly start adding your arms until you are driving them strong. You will immediately feel the twisting go away and your body fall into a smooth, stress-free movement. This is why proper arm drive is important. You want to remember, especially on sprints, to drive your arms parallel to your legs, thinking of them both on the same railroad tracks. The bonus when you do this is the forces meet to balance each other right in your core, giving you an amazing abdominal workout with every step. I always tell people the fastest way to having a six-pack is running. You're burning fat fast while you are constantly working those ab muscles. It's doubling down on your belly area. Be careful, however, to not over-swing your arms in excitement of getting that six-pack. Nice, relaxed hands should not reach and extend past your shoulders—no picking apples when you're running! Your arms will naturally drive in proportion to the force being created by your legs. So, good arm swing means awesome definition in your upper body, and a nice, tight tummy.

## KEY POINTS FROM CHAPTER 7

- For better form, don't run too close to the front of your treadmill.

- Heel-first striking is okay for slow speeds such as walking and jogging, but faster speeds require a forefoot strike to lessen impact.

- Be careful to not overstride when sprinting, and remember to shorten stride on steep hills.

- Maintain runner's tilt, avoiding sitting back on your hips when fatigued.

- Avoid swinging your arms side to side across your center-line. Keeping a nice parallel arm-to-leg drive is important for healthy running and a better body.

## Chapter 8

# INJURIES AND LIMITATIONS

Everything about the way you run tells part of your story. We are now able to identify people with gait recognition technology, based completely on the unique way each of us walks. The way we walk, jog, and run is influenced by our injuries and limitations. We all have them, and they make us unique. The workouts in this book truly are designed for everyone for that very reason. Regardless of your age, limiting factors, or nagging injuries from your past, everything in this book is scalable to fit your circumstances. The great thing about the treadmill is that it is a safe and controlled environment to explore the limits and capabilities of your own circumstances. We are all in this together, and we must all keep moving forward.

### WE ALL HAVE SCARS

*Every time I tie my shoelaces, I see this long white scar on my left shin. And every time I see it, I am reminded that none of us is invincible, that even the strongest of us have had injuries or are limited by factors outside of our control.*

*My only significant injury came in the middle of my college track career. It was an entire year before the brutal NCAA finals I mentioned in the speed chapter. It was January of 2002 in Indianapolis, Indiana. It was the cold indoor season, so the tracks were small (half the size of an outdoor track) and injuries were not uncommon. This particular meet was at the Butler University track, one of my favorites. It was one of the fastest indoor tracks in the country, and I was obsessed with the fact that it had banked curves (most indoor tracks are flat, but premium tracks have banked ends that have a catapulting effect, helping you zip around the turns quickly). I always ran well on Butler's track . . . with the exception of this one time.*

*I had finally begun to run some pretty respectable times for the indoor 800-meter dash, my coach had noticed, and I was finding myself thrust into top heats, with some very fast Division 1 runners and even some pros. I remember checking the list of runners for this particular race and shaking my head in disbelief that I was about to race them. I had a plan, though. With little chance of beating the top three guys, I was going to use them, stay with them, to at least run a new Personal Best. I was feeling good— this was going to be my fastest 800-meter dash ever.*

*At the starting line I stared intently at the shoulders of the guy I had planned to stay with. Bang! The gun went off so quickly it startled me. The indoor 800-meter race is unique in that it is the fastest event in running where runners start in separate lanes but eventually share one inside lane. So there I was, sticking to my plan, right on his shoulders sitting in fourth position. We ran very fast, and I remember feeling surprised that I was holding pace with the top dogs of the 800-meter dash. And then I started to feel brave—maybe I could even pick off one of these guys. Oh, how I still remember that electricity in my veins as I considered making that bold move. That will show my coach how much I am improving!*

*Unfortunately, I never got the opportunity. As we made the third turn I saw in a split second a strange movement come from one of the Indiana racers in the front. I didn't learn this until later, but as he was making his turn into the curve, he leaned so far into the inside bank of the track, he whacked his shoulder on a steel post. And from there it was a domino effect. He stumbled wildly, and the second guy crashed into him, and the third guy put out his hands trying not to smash into him, and then there was me. There was no time to move around, and so I smashed into the back of the guy in front of me. And like a bolt of lightning hitting my leg, someone's razor-sharp spikes connected with my shin and in one swift movement tore open my lower leg.*

*Like a ten-car pileup on the freeway, bodies cartwheeled through the air. The oohs and aahs from the crowd, the thumps of bodies hitting the track, creating the distinct smell of burnt skin as runners skidded across the unforgiving rubber. It was an absolute disaster.*

We all get hurt at some point in our lives. Whether it's falling on the track, a car accident, a slip on the ice, or having a little too much fun on the dance floor, we will all eventually deal with some injury. Ironically, most injured treadmill runners do not get injured running, but doing something else, and just notice it during a run. Hopefully these limitations are temporary, but sometimes they remain with us for the rest of our lives. Regardless of what injury or limitation you may be dealing with, the treadmill can be an unexpected ally and friend in your recovery on your quest to keep moving as best you can.

## Special Conditions

### Physical Injuries

It is hardly a coincidence that nearly every physical therapy rehabilitation facility has a treadmill. The treadmill has the unique ability to work at nearly any pace, any incline, for as much or as little time as you need it to. It is also one of the only ways that physicians, physical therapists, and coaches can monitor you, correct movements, and help guide you to a safe and speedy recovery. Again, because the treadmill is a giant computer, it has the ability to help monitor progression, which is key to overcoming a plaguing injury.

If you are coming back from a surgery or a pregnancy, or are on the mend from a sports injury, the treadmill is a safe and effective place to walk, jog, and eventually run your way toward recovery.

### Orthopedic Limitations

The greatest benefit of using a method like BITE is that it becomes scalable. It was specifically designed to be. I have coached this method to people with a broad spectrum of limitations and conditions. For years, I have helped coach a mother of three with an entirely fused spine. I have seen her limitations, but I have also seen her do remarkable things on the treadmill, moving and listening to her body in a safe, challenging, yet still effective way. Nothing breaks my heart more than to see someone discarded or left out because a workout is not scalable for his or her circumstances. Remember, the speeds you use in this book are entirely formulated to work around *your* best speed, whatever that may be. Walkers can do every workout in the book and reap the same benefits as their slightly faster counterparts. It will also inspire and re-energize those with permanent limitations, helping them discover a new excitement for health and fitness. Because *The Ultimate Treadmill Workout* is the most formulated and mathematical running model ever created for the treadmill, it ensures that everyone fits into the equation.

> As long as you can walk, you can do any workout in this book.

### Pregnancy and Postpartum

As with everything in fitness, your doctor should have the last "professional" word on your ability to work out. I have coached dozens and dozens of women straight through their pregnancies, but they have always been cleared to do cardio.

I always recommend that any woman who is early in her pregnancy, especially in the first 4–6 weeks, dial back her running or not run at all. Most doctors will give a green light to resume a more rigorous workout when you begin the second trimester, which is also the trimester where I have observed the greatest consistency and results in running. I have seen women do extraordinary things, keeping the body in the best shape possible. Every pregnant woman I have worked with through her pregnancy has come back later saying that this type of running made all the

> Your doctor must clear you to do walking/running workouts. Do not begin a new fitness regimen without first consulting your physician.

difference in a healthy, speedy labor, and a rapid return to her pre-baby body. Just remember, a pregnancy is not the time to try to lose weight, but rather to stay strong and healthy. Gone is the idea (unfortunately often stemming from male opinion) that women need to sit home with their feet up. Not only are women incredibly strong during their pregnancy, but there is also an abundance of research and support for the health benefits of keeping active while pregnant.

Just like when running outside, keep it safe and keep it steady. Although the "movement" of running has little chance of hurting an unborn baby, you still have to take care of your own body. Be sure to stay hydrated! That little bundle of joy is also a little bundle of extra weight, so it will take a little extra work for your muscles to keep you moving. Always have a full water bottle when you step on a treadmill, and take small sips of water throughout the entire workout. If you are someone who has a tendency to not drink enough water, make a point to take a sip of water during every recovery. It gives you something to look forward to during the interval. Also remember, if you are going to continue to do cardio through your pregnancy, you need to up your daily calorie intake. If you pick up the intensity of your cardio in the second trimester, aim for an additional 300 calories per day and up to 500 in the third trimester. Your baby needs you to keep your body weight up,

*If you weren't a runner before pregnancy, wait. Now is not the time to introduce new fitness programs your body may not be prepared to handle.*

and don't worry, these extra calories are going to be used if you are active. Michelle Ulrich, a registered dietitian who works with pregnant athletes, reminds women that these extra calories should be rich in folic acid, calcium, iron, and fiber.

Pregnancy is not the time to learn how to become a runner. If you haven't run before, your body is going to go through changes and adaptations it has not experienced before. Being pregnant puts a lot of stress on your body. If running is brand new to you, your body is going to need time to change and adapt to this new workout environment. It is not likely to be able to do so properly or safely if your body is already coping with an entirely different stress. Walking, as long as it is cleared by your physician, is fine on a treadmill, but again, it is not the right time to learn how to become a world-class treadmill runner.

If you were a moderate to frequent runner before you got pregnant, and you are cleared to run, then this method of running is perfect for you. I have had countless female runners find this method of running safe, easy to modify, and exciting enough to curb their running craving. Most doctors and professionals agree that a safe amount of running while pregnant leads to a healthy pregnancy, and an extremely fast recovery postpartum.

I tell all my postpartum clients to be patient with returning to running. There are some stresses on the body postpartum that many women don't think of. Other than regaining core strength there are other things to watch out for. Many women experience small stress fractures in their toes or feet postpartum. Don't forget that the little mini-you who just entered the world took some of your bone density with her. Running, especially fast running, requires a push-off on the little bones in your toes. If those little bones aren't at their best, too much pressure can cause nasty little hairline cracks known as stress fractures. I believe it's perfectly fine

*Postpartum time to return to treadmill running is about 4–6 weeks.*

to return to walking, speed walking, etc., but I always advise a gradual build to around week 6 when it is much safer to start adding back a little more intensity. The timeline to return to running is extremely varied and should be specific to your pregnancy and circumstances. If you have had a cesarean section, for example, you should not be doing *any* running or abdominal work, regardless of how light, for at least 6 weeks postpartum. You may be able to safely do some light walking 3–6 weeks postpartum, but running, because of its intense core engagement, should not happen for at least 6 weeks. If you have had a natural childbirth with no complications you will likely be able to return to light running 2–3 weeks before someone who has had a C-section. If you have not had a stress fracture, it is not something you want to mess with. The great news is that if you stayed active and especially if you ran through part of your pregnancy, you are likely to get that body back quickly. I hear so many of my gals come back after pregnancy and tell me their bodies bounced back and they are in even better shape than they were before they got pregnant. Hard to believe, I know, but I've seen it with my own eyes. In college I raced with a young woman named Mandi Zemba. She was a quiet, shy runner and, like me, hailed from the strange land of the Upper Peninsula of Michigan. She was the most modest runner I have ever met in my life, which was so unexpected, because she is the most decorated student-athlete in the history of Grand Valley State University. She is one of the biggest badasses in college running history. What has always stayed with me was not that she was an eight-time NCAA National Champion, or a thirteen-time NCAA All-American, but that she accomplished so much of this after being pregnant and having a child,

*Note to my gentlemen: Postpartum return for husbands is 0 days, just in case you're wondering!*

right in the middle of her college track career! I saw in her the effect running had on a healthy pregnancy, and how it allowed her to recover and get back to the body and stellar career she had as an athlete.

I'm fortunate that I do not have an orthopedic limitation (although my friends seem to think my dancing skills prove otherwise). But I have been injured, and I have had to take time to recover, and I absolutely have had to use the treadmill to do so. My first injury did happen on the track. Although it was many years ago the scar is a constant reminder of the moment I lay tangled in a mess of bruised runners. I do remember also that the adrenaline in my body got me back to my feet, and with claw marks and a gushing leg I started limping toward the finish line. About half of us ended up finishing the race, although it looked more like the finish of a *Walking Dead* episode. And though it wasn't fair and square, I did beat the guy who was in front of me! He didn't get up and finish, but hey, a win is a win right?

## Chapter 9

# EARN IT!

In a world of ever-increasing climate change, crowded streets, and busier schedules, the treadmill might just be the most useful machine in the new age of urban running. It doesn't have to be boring, or painful, or scary. It can be a loyal partner, there to help you get the most out of this one spectacular life. With the use of this book, it is my sincere hope that you will find a path to becoming a stronger, safer, and more motivated runner. Conquering the perfect run is an experience like no other.

A few years ago, I found myself standing in front of a table of workout books. I was blinded by the same message, over and over. Promises. It was all there, the shortest workout in the world, the most fun workout in the world, the most bizarre, trendy, and the biggest shortcuts ever. I am by no means passing any judgment on any of these workouts, but rather telling you what was missing. We as fitness professionals often trip over ourselves to create the next new craze, the coolest new machine, or the most addictive new way to workout. I stared at that table and realized we have officially reached a tipping point in human health and fitness. We have forgotten. We have run so far, pun intended, from the foundations of what makes us strong, fit, lean, and energized beings. I realized at that moment the greatest innovation I could ever offer in fitness is narrating the return of the run, a return to the foundation of everything we have ever created in fitness. This book is more than a bunch of great workouts; it is a story to remind us that if we take a step back from all the craziness, and find the most effective way to do what we already know how to do, we can become unstoppable.

Engineers have created treadmills that runners before us could have only dreamed of. There has never been a better time to improve, whether you are a walker, a jogger, or a professional athlete. I remind you one last time, however, that you must make the choice to do this work. This is the most powerful message I can share with you. People dislike running for one singular reason—they don't want to do the work. I want you to be better than that. I want you to not be afraid or have excuses, or be surrounded by distractions. The balanced running workouts in this book can and will change your life, but you have to let them and you have to earn it. I offer you no gimmicks, no shortcuts, and no bullshit (sorry, but I mean it). The moment you accept this and make this choice, you will begin to love running and all of its gifts. And when the work gets tough and you feel the treadmill howling below you, take a deep breath and remember my promise to you. Conquer the run, lose yourself in the run, and in that moment you cross the finish line you will feel so strong, so empowered, and ultimately, so proud of your worth. Very few things in life can give you that power. And that, my friends, is everything.

# PART TWO

# THE TREADMILL WORKOUT

## Chapter 10

# THE WORKOUTS

Now that you have all the tools to be a more informed and inspired runner, it's time to get to work. Here are the basics you need to get started.

## Choosing Your Starting Speed—Plug and Play

At the beginning of each run I will tell you exactly how far below your top 1-minute Personal Best to begin. Remember, your PB references the fastest you think you can go for 1 minute *at the end* of a workout. It doesn't matter your ability; as long as you do that one piece of math to decide your starting speed, the run is guaranteed to work. For success in any interval workout you must assess your own ability.

This book is specifically designed as a "plug and play" format. You must plug in your starting speed on your table as a reference, and fill in any changes of speed so you'll always know what speed you should be on. This method of choosing a starting speed is a signature of my method and is critical in creating your own success. I have included an example speed in each workout so you can visualize the changes in speed as they occur. It is only a reference and does not mean that is your speed. As I told you in the beginning of this book, if you want easy, brainless workouts that put you in a category so you don't have to do any thinking for yourself, this book is not for you. If you want the best treadmill workouts in the world, the same workouts taught in the most popular treadmill classes across the country, then this is the way it's done.

You will learn your own Personal Best after just one workout, but to get you started, here is a reminder of ranges most people will fall into.

## Personal Best (1 Minute)

- **4–6 mph**—This PB range works well for people who are new to running or who have physical limitations.

- **6–8 mph**—This PB range is for those who run occasionally, with some experience doing interval training.

- **8–10 mph**—This PB is for those who consider themselves experienced and avid runners, regularly do interval training on treadmills, or run occasional road races.

- **10 mph and up**—This PB range is mostly for those at a high level of run conditioning and competitive runners.

### Reading Your Workout

All workouts are designed on one to three pages with each segment on its own page so you can always keep your workout in your line of sight. Knowing where the workout is going is key to your success, so read it over and become familiar with the flow of each unique workout. Don't skip this step, as being familiar with the run is extremely healthy for your mind and will ensure you maximize your time and efforts in each workout. You have to make the choice to take back the understanding and control of your workout.

### Using Your Treadmill

Here are some tips to remember when using your treadmill. I never recommend speeding up and stepping on a fast-moving treadmill. It's lazy and not safe. Your body is designed to accelerate, so let it. Also be sure you aren't holding onto the treadmill while running. If you can't run without holding on, slow down.

- Lead time—speed up about 10 seconds before the start of every interval.
- Never speed up the treadmill and then step on.
- Program your top speeds if your treadmill has the capability.
- If at home, keep little fingers away from the tread while you are working out.

### Timing

Stay on top of your timing. Whether you are using the clock on the treadmill or you are using a timer on your watch, pay attention to timing. It can sneak up on you quickly. Remember, recoveries are not negotiable. If it is a 1-minute recovery, it must be 1 minute. There is no built-in timer for this book on purpose. Part of what makes this method of running so effective is that it takes away the very shortcuts that can make running on a treadmill boring and mindless. Getting used to the timer, or the clock on your treadmill, is the best way to stay on time. This is a powerful mind exercise as well, requiring you to do some timing math. For example, if the clock on your treadmill says 1:30 and you are starting a 90-second interval, you know you have to run until the clock says 3:00 (adding 90 seconds to 1:30). Some will need a little more practice than others, but I promise you, the effort is absolutely worth it. I also highly recommend you invest in an inexpensive sports watch with a timer, but you could even use the timer on your phone or a stopwatch. However you feel most comfortable keeping track of time, and what works best for you, is ideal. You will become your own coach. And although I wish I could be there with you every time to tell you when to start and when to stop, learning to be your own best coach is one of the most rewarding, addicting, and effective ways to become a better, smarter, and stronger runner.

When the mind is engaged as well as the body, you become empowered to achieve greatness. This is what makes running so great. Become your own master of timing! If timing on one of the more complex intervals gets away from you, don't stress. The beauty of these workouts is that you will benefit and enjoy doing the same run many times, each time becoming more masterful of its timing.

### Stretching—Warm Up and Cool Down

After a few minutes of walking or jogging, you should always go through a brief period of dynamic or active stretching off the treadmill. Static stretches (or holding stretches) are not as safe or effective as active stretches. Begin with gentle, active stretches, which warm up the muscles and tissues of the body by using controlled movements. Slowly rotating your arm in a giant circle at your side is an example of an active stretch. These stretches should always be done before any of the workouts in this book. Butt kicks, high knees, hip rotations, skating side lunges, shoulder rolls—these are examples of dynamic stretches. Don't forget the upper body is just as important in a run as the lower. Although no workouts start with a sprint, they do start fast enough to demand a good warm-up.

Personally, I think the best thing to do after a few minutes of cooling down is to use a foam roller. If you don't have a foam roller, get one! They do wonders in releasing leftover energy and tension in the muscles, ligaments, and tendons. You've probably seen this long, solid tube in the gym or being carried around under someone's arm. Foam rolling accomplishes what is known as myofascial release and has long been the special trick for elite athletes in their rest and recoveries. It works to loosen and lengthen tissue by slowly kneading the muscles. The pressure from the kneading releases the tight connective tissue (fascia) around the muscles, relaxes tendons, and increases blood flow. Using a foam roller in a warm up is also an extremely effective tool for those who have very limited flexibility or have a history of muscle pulls. Finding the time to use a roller before and after a run is time very well spent. One of the leading companies for recovery products is TriggerPoint, which does a fantastic job providing educational workshops and resources on how to best use this form of restorative therapy.

If you want to also add in some more traditional static stretches, the best time is after the cool-down.

## Chapter 11

# THREE-WEEK KICK-START

Welcome to the introductory workouts for your first Balanced Interval Training Experience! These workouts will gradually build in length and complexity, to ensure no matter your ability, you will create a solid base and be well prepared to conquer the Six-Week Running Revolution. You'll tackle three runs each week, so I recommend that you space out the runs as best you can to fit your schedule, with at least 1 day between workouts. After you read the breakdown, the tables will make it clear and easy to understand what you'll be doing. Take a deep breath and be prepared to have an entirely new relationship with your treadmill.

# WEEK 1

This first week you will work on three relatively short, 20-minute runs.

## RUN 1—THE SIMPLE 60

This is the perfect introduction to the program: a series of 60-second intervals in two segments. You'll work on building incline, then work on taking it away and replacing it with added speed.

### Segment 1

*How To:* Start **1.5 mph under your 1-minute PB**. Use the Suggested Personal Best Speed Ranges in Chapter 4 to determine your starting speed. This will be the first time learning what your PB is, so don't worry if you feel a little off. You'll have a much better idea of your PB after this first run. In this segment you will keep the same light, fast speed every time, but increase incline gradually.

| Interval | Speed | Your Speed | Incline | Recovery (all 0%) |
|---|---|---|---|---|
| 60 seconds | −1.5 mph from PB Ex: 6.5 | | 0% | 1 minute moderate recovery |
| 60 seconds | Same speed | | 1% | 1 minute moderate recovery |
| 60 seconds | Same speed | | 2% | 1 minute moderate recovery |
| 60 seconds | Same speed | | 3% | 2 minutes complete recovery |

## Segment 2

*How To:* Start **on your segment 1 speed**, repeating the last interval in segment 1. Then you'll add 0.5 mph to each interval as the incline goes back down. This run will help you assess what your 1-minute fastest goal speed should be. You should feel maxed out on your last interval.

| Interval | Speed | Your Speed | Incline | Recovery (all 0%) |
|---|---|---|---|---|
| 60 seconds | Last speed Ex: 6.5 | | 3% | 1 minute moderate recovery |
| 60 seconds | +0.5 mph Ex: 7 | | 2% | 1 minute moderate recovery |
| 60 seconds | +0.5 mph Ex: 7.5 | | 1% | 1 minute moderate recovery |
| 60 seconds | +0.5 mph Ex: 8 | | 0% | Cool down |

# WEEK 1—Run 1

Date: _____

Start Speed: _____

PB Goal: _____

Average Recovery Speed: _____

Mileage: _____

Notes:

_____

_____

_____

_____

_____

_____

_____

_____

_____

_____

_____

_____

_____

_____

# WEEK 1

## RUN 2—STUCK

This run is a pyramid in two segments. You climb the pyramid making the intervals shorter, then you climb back down making them longer again. The reason it's called Stuck is because once you reach the speed at the top of the pyramid, you are stuck with that speed all the way back down. Good luck!

## Segment 1

*How To:* Start **1 mph under your 1-minute PB**. Notice you will actually add more than 1 mph, but it's because you are ending on a shorter 30-second interval, which should be a little better than a 1-minute PB. Simply add 0.5 mph to each interval and drop the incline as noted.

| Interval | Speed | Your Speed | Incline | Recovery (all 0%) |
|---|---|---|---|---|
| 60 seconds | −1 mph from PB Ex: 7 | | 5% | 1 minute moderate recovery |
| 50 seconds | +0.5 mph Ex: 7.5 | | 3% | 1 minute moderate recovery |
| 40 seconds | +0.5 mph Ex: 8 | | 1% | 1 minute moderate recovery |
| 30 seconds | +0.5 mph Ex: 8.5 | | 0% | 2 minutes complete recovery |

## Segment 2

*How To:* Simply **start where you left off**, repeating the last interval you did in segment 1, but now doing it on a 3% incline. From there, you will have the challenge of being "stuck" on the same top speed as the intervals get longer, all on a 3% incline, until you arrive back on the 60-second interval.

| Interval | Speed | Your Speed | Incline | Recovery (all 0%) |
|----------|-------|------------|---------|-------------------|
| 30 seconds | Last speed Ex: 8.5 | | 3% | 1 minute moderate recovery |
| 40 seconds | Same speed | | 3% | 1 minute moderate recovery |
| 50 seconds | Same speed | | 3% | 1 minute moderate recovery |
| 60 seconds | Same speed | | 3% | Cool down |

# WEEK 1—Run 2

Date: _____

Start Speed: _____

PB Goal: _____

Average Recovery Speed: _____

Mileage: _____

Notes:

_____

_____

_____

_____

_____

_____

_____

_____

_____

_____

_____

_____

# WEEK 1

## RUN 3—EVIL TWIN

It's time to start getting a little more interesting, so for this run you'll do an interval on a 0% (nice twin) but then do the exact same interval on an incline (evil twin). This is a smaller version of a run in the 6-week challenge to look forward to.

### Segment 1

*How To:* Start **1.5 mph under your 1-minute PB**. You'll do three sets of twins, with each set getting a little faster but shorter. Once you add speed to an interval (nice twin), you maintain that new speed on the incline (evil twin).

| Interval | Speed | Your Speed | Incline | Recovery (all 0%) |
|---|---|---|---|---|
| 60 seconds | −1.5 mph from PB Ex: 6.5 | | 0% | 1 minute moderate recovery |
| 60 seconds | Same speed | | 4% | 1 minute moderate recovery |
| 45 seconds | +0.5 mph Ex: 7 | | 0% | 1 minute moderate recovery |
| 45 seconds | Same speed | | 4% | 1 minute moderate recovery |
| 30 seconds | +0.5 mph Ex: 7.5 | | 0% | 1 minute moderate recovery |
| 30 seconds | Same speed | | 4% | 2 minutes complete recovery |

### Segment 2

*How To:* There is a surprise challenge here. You must now repeat the first segment but start **at the speed you ended segment 1**. Basically, you are starting 1 mph faster than you started segment 1. Incline is a little less on the evil-twin interval to balance the increase in speeds. Note that you *will* exceed your 1-minute PB as the intervals fall below 1 minute.

| Interval | Speed | Your Speed | Incline | Recovery (all 0%) |
|---|---|---|---|---|
| 60 seconds | Last speed Ex: 7.5 | | 0% | 1 minute moderate recovery |
| 60 seconds | Same speed | | 3% | 1 minute moderate recovery |
| 45 seconds | +0.5 mph Ex: 8 | | 0% | 1 minute moderate recovery |
| 45 seconds | Same speed | | 3% | 1 minute moderate recovery |
| 30 seconds | +0.5 mph Ex: 8.5 | | 0% | 1 minute moderate recovery |
| 30 seconds | Same speed | | 3% | Cool down |

# WEEK 1—Run 3

Date: _____

Start Speed: _____

PB Goal: _____

Average Recovery Speed: _____

Mileage: _____

Notes:

_____

_____

_____

_____

_____

_____

_____

_____

_____

_____

_____

_____

_____

_____

# WEEK 2

This week we are going to lengthen your workouts by 10 minutes. It may not sound like much, but increasing your runs to 30 minutes is going to start challenging your focus and stamina. It's also time to start showing you how to challenge recoveries to increase your burn and make you stronger.

## RUN 4—RECOVERY CLIMB

This run is all about the intervals getting faster, and then teaching you one of three ways the BITE method will challenge your recovery.

## Segment 1

*How To:* Start **1 mph under your 1-minute PB**. There is no incline in this segment, but don't worry; it's coming! Simply add 0.2 mph to each interval.

| Interval | Speed | Your Speed | Incline | Recovery (all 0%) |
|---|---|---|---|---|
| 60 seconds | −1 mph from PB Ex: 7 | | 0% | 1 minute moderate recovery |
| 60 seconds | +0.2 mph Ex: 7.2 | | 0% | 1 minute moderate recovery |
| 60 seconds | +0.2 mph Ex: 7.4 | | 0% | 1 minute moderate recovery |
| 60 seconds | +0.2 mph Ex: 7.6 | | 0% | 1 minute moderate recovery |
| 60 seconds | +0.2 mph Ex: 7.8 | | 0% | 1 minute moderate recovery |
| 60 seconds | +0.2 mph Ex: 8 | | 0% | 2 minutes complete recovery |

### Segment 2

*How To:* Now you must try to **hold your top speed** for each of these 1-minute intervals but with a recovery that gets steeper each time. Note: you must try to add your incline immediately after the interval ends at the start of the recovery, or you'll miss it, and the great challenge before you.

| Interval | Speed | Your Speed | Incline | Recovery |
|---|---|---|---|---|
| 60 seconds | Last speed Ex: 8 | | 0% interval; 3% recovery | 1 minute moderate recovery at 3% incline |
| 60 seconds | Same speed | | 0% interval; 4% recovery | 1 minute same recovery speed at 4% incline |
| 60 seconds | Same speed | | 0% interval; 5% recovery | 1 minute same recovery speed at 5% incline |
| 60 seconds | Same speed | | 0% interval; 6% recovery | 1 minute same recovery speed at 6% incline |
| 60 seconds | Same speed | | 0% interval; 7% recovery | 1 minute same recovery speed at 7% incline |
| 60 seconds | Same speed | | 0% interval | Cool down |

# WEEK 2—Run 4

Date: _____

Start Speed: _____

PB Goal: _____

Average Recovery Speed: _____

Mileage: _____

Notes:

_____

_____

_____

_____

_____

_____

_____

_____

_____

_____

_____

_____

_____

_____

_____

# WEEK 2

## RUN 5—RECOVERY SHRINK

This run is about the incredible shrinking recovery. First we will get the intervals faster, and then you'll get a taste of having your recovery shrink in time, which is another one of the three ways to challenge recovery. This one is all about the clock, so stay on it!

## Segment 1

*How To:* Start **2 mph under your 1-minute PB**. Your incline will go down with every addition of speed. It will get fast quick!

| Interval | Speed | Your Speed | Incline | Recovery (all 0%) |
|---|---|---|---|---|
| 60 seconds | −2 mph from PB Ex: 6 | | 5% | 1 minute moderate recovery |
| 60 seconds | +0.4 mph Ex: 6.4 | | 4% | 1 minute moderate recovery |
| 60 seconds | +0.4 mph Ex: 6.8 | | 3% | 1 minute moderate recovery |
| 60 seconds | +0.4 mph Ex: 7.2 | | 2% | 1 minute moderate recovery |
| 60 seconds | +0.4 mph Ex: 7.6 | | 1% | 1 minute moderate recovery |
| 60 seconds | +0.4 mph Ex: 8 | | 0% | 2–3 minutes complete recovery |

### Segment 2

*How To:* You'll grow the same total amount of speed as segment 1 (adding +0.5 mph instead of +0.4 mph because there's one less interval). However, this time the incline is 0% because your recovery shrinks by 10 seconds every time. Stay focused on the clock and the challenge will be eye opening. Be sure to watch the clock closely!

| Interval | Speed | Your Speed | Incline | Recovery (all 0%) |
|---|---|---|---|---|
| 60 seconds | −2 mph from PB Ex: 6 | | 0% | 60 seconds moderate recovery |
| 60 seconds | +0.5 mph Ex: 6.5 | | 0% | 50 seconds moderate recovery |
| 60 seconds | +0.5 mph Ex: 7 | | 0% | 40 seconds moderate recovery |
| 60 seconds | +0.5 mph Ex: 7.5 | | 0% | 30 seconds moderate recovery |
| 60 seconds | +0.5 mph Ex: 8 | | 0% | Cool down |

*THE ULTIMATE TREADMILL WORKOUT*

# WEEK 2—Run 5

Date: _____

Start Speed: _____

PB Goal: _____

Average Recovery Speed: _____

Mileage: _____

Notes:

_____

_____

_____

_____

_____

_____

_____

_____

_____

_____

_____

_____

_____

_____

_____

# WEEK 2

## RUN 6—RECOVERY SPEED

Now I will show you how to use speed to challenge a recovery. First you will build your speed on the interval. Then in the last segment you'll take your interval speed back down, but you will pick up your recovery speed for another surprising challenge.

# WEEK 2—Run 6

### Segment 1

*How To:* Start **1 mph under your 1-minute PB**. We are back to 1-minute intervals, growing 1 full point faster by your last one. You should be getting close to pinning down what your best 1-minute should be. There is just a little bit of incline here to help warm you up.

| Interval | Speed | Your Speed | Incline | Recovery (all 0%) |
|---|---|---|---|---|
| 60 seconds | −1 mph from PB Ex: 7 | | 2% | 1 minute moderate recovery |
| 60 seconds | +0.2 mph Ex: 7.2 | | 2% | 1 minute moderate recovery |
| 60 seconds | +0.2 mph Ex: 7.4 | | 2% | 1 minute moderate recovery |
| 60 seconds | +0.2 mph Ex: 7.6 | | 2% | 1 minute moderate recovery |
| 60 seconds | +0.2 mph Ex: 7.8 | | 2% | 1 minute moderate recovery |
| 60 seconds | +0.2 mph Ex: 8 | | 2% | 2 minutes complete recovery |

## Segment 2

*How To:* Start **at the speed where you left off in segment 1**. Now you'll go back down in speed until you arrive back where you started in segment 1. The difference, however, is that every time you take away interval speed you'll have to add recovery speed (−0.2 from interval but +0.3 to recovery). Your first recovery speed should be exactly **3 mph** under your interval speed. It's the ultimate tug of war between interval speed and recovery speed. Be sure to fill in the Your Recovery Speed column that I've added for you. You won't get lost if you do that.

| Interval | Speed | Your Speed | Your Recovery Speed | Incline | Recovery (all 0%) |
|----------|-------|------------|---------------------|---------|-------------------|
| 60 seconds | Last speed Ex: 8 | | | 0% | 1 minute −3 mph from interval speed Ex: 5 |
| 60 seconds | −0.2 mph Ex: 7.8 | | | 0% | 1 minute +0.3 mph to last recovery speed Ex: 5.3 |
| 60 seconds | −0.2 mph Ex: 7.6 | | | 0% | 1 minute +0.3 mph to last recovery speed Ex: 5.6 |
| 60 seconds | −0.2 mph Ex: 7.4 | | | 0% | 1 minute +0.3 mph to last recovery speed Ex: 5.9 |
| 60 seconds | −0.2 mph Ex: 7.2 | | | 0% | 1 minute +0.3 mph to last recovery speed Ex: 6.2 |
| 60 seconds | −0.2 mph Ex: 7 | | | 0% | Cool down |

# WEEK 2—Run 6

Date: _____

Start Speed: _____

PB Goal: _____

Average Recovery Speed: _____

Mileage: _____

Notes:

_____

_____

_____

_____

_____

_____

_____

_____

_____

_____

_____

_____

# WEEK 3

Novice runners should now be feeling more confident, and strong runners should be itching for the bigger runs. This is the final step in building a strong, healthy foundation, and as a bonus, we are about to rev up the fat burning in a big way. You conquer these and you can conquer anything!

## RUN 7—BUILD-A-BURN

We will now introduce the 90-second interval. It's never as much fun as a 30-second dash, but with a little discipline you will gain endurance, increase your fat burn, and start to see results you never imagined. This is a three-segment run, doing a set of 60s, a set of 30s, and finally, a set of 90s.

# WEEK 3—Run 7

## Segment 1

*How To:* Start **2 mph under your 1-minute PB**. Although you won't add any speed on these 1-minute intervals, you will be adding incline.

| Interval | Speed | Your Speed | Incline | Recovery (all 0%) |
|---|---|---|---|---|
| 60 seconds | −1 mph from PB Ex: 7 | | 1% | 1 minute moderate recovery |
| 60 seconds | Same speed | | 2% | 1 minute moderate recovery |
| 60 seconds | Same speed | | 3% | 1 minute moderate recovery |
| 60 seconds | Same speed | | 4% | 1 minute moderate recovery |
| 60 seconds | Same speed | | 5% | 1 minute moderate recovery |
| 60 seconds | Same speed | | 6% | 2 minutes complete recovery |

### Segment 2

*How To:* Start **on the ending speed from segment 1**. You'll pick up where you left off on incline and this time go back down in incline as you start to add speed. Note: you will exceed your PB because it's only a 30-second sprint.

| Interval | Speed | Your Speed | Incline | Recovery (all 0%) |
|---|---|---|---|---|
| 30 seconds | Last speed Ex: 7 | | 6% | 1 minute moderate recovery |
| 30 seconds | +0.3 mph Ex: 7.3 | | 5% | 1 minute moderate recovery |
| 30 seconds | +0.3 mph Ex: 7.6 | | 4% | 1 minute moderate recovery |
| 30 seconds | +0.3 mph Ex: 7.9 | | 3% | 1 minute moderate recovery |
| 30 seconds | +0.3 mph Ex: 8.2 | | 2% | 1 minute moderate recovery |
| 30 seconds | +0.3 mph Ex: 8.5 | | 1% | 2 minutes complete recovery |

### Segment 3

*How To:* Start all of these intervals **on the same speed from segment 1**. Now you will combine work from segment 1 with segment 2. After 60 seconds you'll add on the 30 seconds with additional speed as noted.

| Interval | | Speed | Your Speed | Incline | Recovery (all 0%) |
|---|---|---|---|---|---|
| (90 seconds) | 60 seconds | Segment 1 speed Ex: 7 | | 0% | 1 minute moderate recovery |
| | 30 seconds | +0.3 mph Ex: 7.3 | | | |
| (90 seconds) | 60 seconds | Same start speed Ex: 7 | | 0% | 1 minute moderate recovery |
| | 30 seconds | +0.6 mph Ex: 7.6 | | | |
| (90 seconds) | 60 seconds | Same start speed Ex: 7 | | 0% | 1 minute moderate recovery |
| | 30 seconds | +0.9 mph Ex: 7.9 | | | |
| (90 seconds) | 60 seconds | Same start speed Ex: 7 | | 0% | 1 minute moderate recovery |
| | 30 seconds | +1.2 mph Ex: 8.2 | | | |
| (90 seconds) | 60 seconds | Same start speed Ex: 7 | | 0% | Cool down |
| | 30 seconds | +1.5 mph Ex: 8.5 | | | |

# WEEK 3—Run 7

Date: _____

Start Speed: _____

PB Goal: _____

Average Recovery Speed: _____

Mileage: _____

Notes:

_____

_____

_____

_____

_____

_____

_____

_____

_____

_____

_____

_____

_____

_____

# WEEK 3

## RUN 8—FARTLEK FOUNDATION

This run shows you a foundational fartlek workout using the BITE method. Fartleks are common in running and essentially stand for speed play.

## Segment 1

*How To:* Choose three speeds to commit to in a cycle. I recommend your easy speed is exactly **3 mph under your 1-minute PB**. Your medium is 1 point faster than that and your fast is 1 point faster than that. Those three speeds do not change in this round. It's important to remember that **your easy minute is your only recovery in this fartlek**. There is no incline, as this allows you to practice the foundation of the cycle effect of a fartlek.

| Interval | Speed | Your Speed | Incline | Recovery (0%) |
|---|---|---|---|---|
| 1 minute Easy | −3 mph from PB Ex: 5 | | 0% | None |
| 1 minute Medium | +1 mph Ex: 6 | | 0% | None |
| 1 minute Fast | +1 mph Ex: 7 | | 0% | None |
| 1 minute Easy | Same Easy Ex: 5 | | 0% | None |
| 1 minute Medium | Same Medium Ex: 6 | | 0% | None |
| 1 minute Fast | Same Fast Ex: 7 | | 0% | None |
| 1 minute Easy | Same Easy Ex: 5 | | 0% | None |
| 1 minute Medium | Same Medium Ex: 6 | | 0% | None |
| 1 minute Fast | Same Fast Ex: 7 | | 0% | 2–3 minute complete recovery |

## Segment 2

*How To:* Now you'll use **the exact same three speeds from segment 1**. You will simply add the paired incline to each speed to experience how a small change in a fartlek adds up quickly. **Remember, your easy interval is your recovery period in this fartlek.**

| Interval | Speed | Your Speed | Incline | Recovery (0%) |
|---|---|---|---|---|
| 1 minute Easy | −3 mph from PB Ex: 5 | | 3% | None |
| 1 minute Medium | +1 mph Ex: 6 | | 2% | None |
| 1 minute Fast | +1 mph Ex: 7 | | 1% | None |
| 1 minute Easy | Same Easy Ex: 5 | | 3% | None |
| 1 minute Medium | Same Medium Ex: 6 | | 2% | None |
| 1 minute Fast | Same Fast Ex: 7 | | 1% | None |
| 1 minute Easy | Same Easy Ex: 5 | | 3% | None |
| 1 minute Medium | Same Medium Ex: 6 | | 2% | None |
| 1 minute Fast | Same Fast Ex: 7 | | 1% | 2–3 minute complete recovery |

### Segment 3

*How To:* Start **with the exact three speeds from segment 2**. Now you will make all three speeds faster with the inclines from segment 2. After the first cycle of Easy, Medium, and Fast, you will add 0.5 mph to each speed. You'll do that twice. And remember, **your easy minute is your only recovery**.

| Interval | Speed | Your Speed | Incline | Recovery (0%) |
| --- | --- | --- | --- | --- |
| 1 minute Easy | −3 mph from PB Ex: 5 | | 3% | None |
| 1 minute Medium | +1 mph Ex: 6 | | 2% | None |
| 1 minute Fast | +1 mph Ex: 7 | | 1% | None |
| 1 minute Easy | Easy +0.5 mph Ex: 5.5 | | 3% | None |
| 1 minute Medium | +1 mph Ex: 6.5 | | 2% | None |
| 1 minute Fast | +1 mph Ex: 7.5 | | 1% | None |
| 1 minute Easy | Easy +1 mph Ex: 6 | | 3% | None |
| 1 minute Medium | +1 mph Ex: 7 | | 2% | None |
| 1 minute Fast | +1 mph Ex: 8 | | 1% | Cool down |

# WEEK 3—Run 8

Date: _____

Start Speed: _____

PB Goal: _____

Average Recovery Speed: _____

Mileage: _____

Notes:

_____

_____

_____

_____

_____

_____

_____

_____

_____

_____

_____

_____

_____

# WEEK 3

## RUN 9—TERRIBLE TWOS

Don't worry; they aren't actually terrible, but they absolutely are all 2-minute intervals, the longest the BITE method will ever prescribe. Okay, maybe they are just a little terrible. It's a two-segment run, one playing with inclines, and the other with speeds. We must all go through the terrible-twos phase of our lives, and so shall we the 2-minute intervals.

## Segment 1

*How To:* Start **2 mph under your 1-minute PB**. The only changes in this segment are the inclines. Make note of where the incline changes during the interval and be sure to stay on top of the changes. Each interval is 2 minutes long and you should have a 1-minute recovery between each interval.

| Interval | | Speed | Your Speed | Incline | Recovery (all 0%) |
|---|---|---|---|---|---|
| (2 minutes) | 1 minute | −2 mph from PB Ex: 6 | | 0% | 1 minute moderate recovery |
| | 30 seconds +% | | | 1% | |
| | 30 seconds +% | | | 3% | |
| (2 minutes) | 1 minute | Same speed | | 0% | 1 minute moderate recovery |
| | 30 seconds +% | | | 2% | |
| | 30 seconds +% | | | 4% | |
| (2 minutes) | 1 minute | Same speed | | 0% | 1 minute moderate recovery |
| | 30 seconds +% | | | 3% | |
| | 30 seconds +% | | | 5% | |
| (2 minutes) | 1 minute | Same speed | | 0% | 1 minute moderate recovery |
| | 30 seconds +% | | | 4% | |
| | 30 seconds +% | | | 6% | |
| (2 minutes) | 1 minute | Same speed | | 0% | 1 minute moderate recovery |
| | 30 seconds +% | | | 5% | |
| | 30 seconds +% | | | 7% | |
| (2 minutes) | 1 minute | Same speed | | 0% | 2 minutes complete recovery |
| | 30 seconds +% | | | 6% | |
| | 30 seconds +% | | | 8% | |

## Segment 2

*How To:* Start all these intervals **on segment 1 speed**. Just like you did with incline, now you will add speed after 1 minute, then again in 30 seconds. It is the last 30 seconds of the interval that will grow and grow, exceeding your PB. Each interval is 2 minutes long and you should have a 1-minute recovery between each interval.

| Interval | | Speed | Your Speed | Incline | Recovery (all 0%) |
|---|---|---|---|---|---|
| (2 minutes) | 1 minute | Last speed Ex: 6 | | 0% | 1 minute easy recovery |
| | 30 seconds | +0.5 Ex: 6.5 | | | |
| | 30 seconds | +0.5 Ex: 7 | | | |
| (2 minutes) | 1 minute | Start speed Ex: 6 | | 0% | 1 minute easy recovery |
| | 30 seconds | +0.5 Ex: 6.5 | | | |
| | 30 seconds | +0.7 Ex: 7.2 | | | |
| (2 minutes) | 1 minute | Start speed Ex: 6 | | 0% | 1 minute easy recovery |
| | 30 seconds | +0.5 Ex: 6.5 | | | |
| | 30 seconds | +0.9 Ex: 7.4 | | | |
| (2 minutes) | 1 minute | Start speed Ex: 6 | | 0% | 1 minute easy recovery |
| | 30 seconds | +0.5 Ex: 6.5 | | | |
| | 30 seconds | +1.1 Ex: 7.6 | | | |
| (2 minutes) | 1 minute | Start speed Ex: 6 | | 0% | 1 minute easy recovery |
| | 30 seconds | +0.5 Ex: 6.5 | | | |
| | 30 seconds | +1.3 Ex: 7.8 | | | |
| (2 minutes) | 1 minute | Start speed Ex: 6 | | 0% | Cool down |
| | 30 seconds | +0.5 Ex: 6.5 | | | |
| | 30 seconds | +1.5 Ex: 8 | | | |

# WEEK 3—Run 9

Date: _____

Start Speed: _____

PB Goal: _____

Average Recovery Speed: _____

Mileage: _____

Notes:

_____

_____

_____

_____

_____

_____

_____

_____

_____

_____

_____

_____

_____

_____

## Chapter 12

# THE SIX-WEEK RUNNING REVOLUTION

This is the exciting, addictive, and highly effective 6-week treadmill program that is certain to help you reach an entirely new level of health and fitness. This step-by-step program will help you shed unwanted weight quickly and safely, and help you become a better runner. These are simply the most amazing treadmill workouts ever. These amazing, easy-to-follow workouts will eradicate the treadmill boredom that turns off so many would-be runners. You will not look at the treadmill or your body the same way after this 6-week transformation.

Make sure you refer back to the tips on getting started throughout Part 1 of the book. You'll conquer three runs per week, so it's important you work out your schedule the best you can for optimal performance. Try to give yourself at least 1 day between workouts. Choose the 3 days each week you will do these workouts, and make the commitment to show up.

It's important that you use your days off wisely. I am a big proponent of weight training on off days, and filling those days with other forms of lower-impact cardio like cycling or swimming. Yoga is also a great complement to running, as it helps deal with some of the tightness one feels from running.

As I said in the beginning of this book, you have to make the choice to bring the work back into your workout. Let this be the moment you bring running back into your life. It won't be easy at first, but it will be one of the most rewarding and empowering experiences of your life. Make the choice, and make it now!

# WEEK 1

In this first week we will start with some foundation runs. You will practice the most common intervals to start, then learn how to perfect incline changes, and finally how to conquer the long 2-minute intervals.

## RUN 1—THE DOUBLE TRIPLE

This is a great first run, as it covers the three most common intervals found in treadmill training; the 30, 60, and 90. We do a 30-second interval, then double that work with a 60, then triple the work by doing a challenging 90-second interval.

### Segment 1

*How To:* Start **2 mph under your 1-minute PB**. This one is about the incline. We will do moderate 30-, 60-, and 90-second intervals all at the same speed and an incline of 4%. The challenge will be holding on to these variables as the interval gets longer and longer. Even though you don't change speed, make a note of your speed in your column for reference. Notice you also get a 90-second recovery after the 90-second interval. You're welcome!

| Interval | Speed | Your Speed | Incline | Recovery (all 0%) |
|---|---|---|---|---|
| 30 seconds | −2 mph from PB Ex: 6 | | 4% | 1 minute walk/jog |
| 60 seconds | Same speed | | 4% | 1 minute walk/jog |
| 90 seconds | Same speed | | 4% | 90 seconds walk/jog |
| 30 seconds | Same speed | | 6% | 1 minute walk/jog |
| 60 seconds | Same speed | | 6% | 1 minute walk/jog |
| 90 seconds | Same speed | | 6% | 1 minute walk/jog |

## Segment 2

*How To:* Start **1 mph faster than segment 1.** Now we will try the same format of 30, 60, 90 but without any incline. The challenge will now be to start on a faster speed and hold that speed as the intervals get longer and longer. Add 1 mph to your speed from segment 1 and fill in your speed column to reference.

| Interval | Speed | Your Speed | Incline | Recovery (all 0%) |
|----------|-------|------------|---------|-------------------|
| 30 seconds | Segment 1 speed +1 mph Ex: 7 | | 0% | 1 minute walk/jog |
| 60 seconds | Same speed | | 0% | 1 minute walk/jog |
| 90 seconds | Same speed | | 0% | 90 seconds walk/jog |
| 30 seconds | +0.5 mph Ex: 7.5 | | 0% | 1 minute walk/jog |
| 60 seconds | Same speed | | 0% | 1 minute walk/jog |
| 90 seconds | Same speed | | 0% | 1 minute walk/jog |

### Segment 3

*How To:* Start **0.5 mph faster than you ended segment 2, which should be your PB**. Finally we attempt to do one more set of 30, 60, 90, but even faster than in segment 2, and with some incline from segment 1. The challenge is to handle the incline *and* speed increase.

| Interval | Speed | Your Speed | Incline | Recovery (all 0%) |
|----------|-------|------------|---------|-------------------|
| 30 seconds | Last speed +0.5 mph Ex: 8 | | 3% | 1 minute walk/jog |
| 60 seconds | Same speed | | 3% | 1 minute walk/jog |
| 90 seconds | Same speed | | 3% | Cool down |

# WEEK 1—Run 1

Date: _____

Start Speed: _____

PB Goal: _____

Average Recovery Speed: _____

Mileage: _____

Notes:

_____

_____

_____

_____

_____

_____

_____

_____

_____

_____

_____

_____

_____

# WEEK 1

## RUN 2—INCLINE PYRAMID

Now that we have become a little more familiar with the 30-, 60-, and 90-second intervals, let's isolate them and focus on doing some repeat intervals with a little incline twist. Very simply, each segment has a different set of interval lengths and will climb and descend a bigger and bigger pyramid of incline.

### Segment 1

*How To:* Start **1 mph under your 1-minute PB**. You will do five 90-second intervals. You'll go down in incline as you add speed, but as you reach the bottom incline (1%) you must take your speed back up the incline.

| Interval | Speed | Your Speed | Incline | Recovery (all 0%) |
|---|---|---|---|---|
| 90 seconds | −1 mph from PB Ex: 7 | | 3% | 1 minute walk/jog |
| 90 seconds | +0.2 mph Ex: 7.2 | | 2% | 1 minute walk/jog |
| 90 seconds | +0.2 mph Ex: 7.4 | | 1% | 1 minute walk/jog |
| 90 seconds | Same speed | | 2% | 1 minute walk/jog |
| 90 seconds | Same speed | | 3% | 2 minute recovery |

## Segment 2

*How To:* Start **0.2 mph faster than you ended segment 1**. You'll do the same format as segment 1 but now with seven 60-second intervals and a pyramid with a slightly steeper incline. Continue filling in your speeds for quick reference.

| Interval | Speed | Your Speed | Incline | Recovery (all 0%) |
|---|---|---|---|---|
| 60 seconds | Last speed +0.2 mph Ex: 7.6 | | 4% | 1 minute walk/jog |
| 60 seconds | +0.2 mph Ex: 7.8 | | 3% | 1 minute walk/jog |
| 60 seconds | +0.2 mph Ex: 8 | | 2% | 1 minute walk/jog |
| 60 seconds | +0.2 mph Ex: 8.2 | | 1% | 1 minute walk/jog |
| 60 seconds | Same speed | | 2% | 1 minute walk/jog |
| 60 seconds | Same speed | | 3% | 1 minute walk/jog |
| 60 seconds | Same speed | | 4% | 2 minute recovery |

## Segment 3

*How To:* Start **0.2 mph faster than you ended segment 2**. This is the same format once again, except we will now do seven 30-second intervals and the incline pyramid starts at its steepest. Note you'll exceed your PB because you end on a shorter 30-second interval.

| Interval | Speed | Your Speed | Incline | Recovery (all 0%) |
|----------|-------|------------|---------|-------------------|
| 30 seconds | Last speed +0.2 mph Ex: 8.4 | | 5% | 1 minute walk/jog |
| 30 seconds | +0.2 mph Ex: 8.6 | | 4% | 1 minute walk/jog |
| 30 seconds | +0.2 mph Ex: 8.8 | | 3% | 1 minute walk/jog |
| 30 seconds | +0.2 mph Ex: 9 | | 2% | 1 minute walk/jog |
| 30 seconds | Same speed | | 3% | 1 minute walk/jog |
| 30 seconds | Same speed | | 4% | 1 minute walk/jog |
| 30 seconds | Same speed | | 5% | Cool down |

Date: _____

Start Speed: _____

PB Goal: _____

Average Recovery Speed: _____

Mileage: _____

Notes:

_____

_____

_____

_____

_____

_____

_____

_____

_____

_____

_____

_____

_____

_____

# WEEK 1

## RUN 3—THE BREAKDOWN

Now it's time to let you experience the maximum of one of the BITE method's guidelines, the longest interval the method prescribes: the 2-minute interval! But to make these long intervals not seem so long we will make several changes within the interval to keep you engaged and alert. A 2-minute interval will help you quickly strengthen your endurance.

## Segment 1

*How To:* Start **1 mph under your 1-minute PB**. A lot happens in these intervals, so follow closely. After 1 minute you will slow down 1 mph, then for the last 30 seconds you will drop your incline to 0%. The starting incline is difficult and eases off slightly before recovery.

| Interval | | Speed | Your Speed | Incline | Recovery (all 0%) |
|---|---|---|---|---|---|
| (2 minutes) | 60 seconds | −1 mph from PB Ex: 7 | | 1% | 1 minute walk/jog |
| | 30 seconds | −1 mph Ex: 6 | | 1% | |
| | 30 seconds | Same speed −% | | 0% | |
| (2 minutes) | 60 seconds | −1 mph from PB Ex: 7 | | 2% | 1 minute walk/jog |
| | 30 seconds | −1 mph Ex: 6 | | 2% | |
| | 30 seconds | Same speed −% | | 0% | |
| (2 minutes) | 60 seconds | −1 mph from PB Ex: 7 | | 3% | 1 minute walk/jog |
| | 30 seconds | −1 mph Ex: 6 | | 3% | |
| | 30 seconds | Same speed −% | | 0% | |
| (2 minutes) | 60 seconds | −1 mph from PB Ex: 7 | | 4% | 1 minute walk/jog |
| | 30 seconds | −1 mph Ex: 6 | | 4% | |
| | 30 seconds | Same speed −% | | 0% | |
| (2 minutes) | 60 seconds | −1 mph from PB Ex: 7 | | 5% | 2 minute recovery |
| | 30 seconds | −1 mph Ex: 6 | | 5% | |
| | 30 seconds | Same speed −% | | 0% | |

### Segment 2

*How To:* Start **0.2 mph faster than you *started* segment 1**. This is a complex run but very effective. Now we will break down five 2-minute intervals with speed. The first 60 seconds of the interval will grow in speed, then you'll always take away 1 mph from that speed, then you'll take away what you added to the beginning. Follow the examples to better understand. You'll end on the same speed every time.

| Interval | | Speed | Your Speed | Incline | Recovery (all 0%) |
|---|---|---|---|---|---|
| (2 minutes) | 60 seconds | First start speed +0.2 mph Ex: 7.2 | | 0% | 1 minute walk/jog |
| | 30 seconds | −1 mph Ex: 6.2 | | | |
| | 30 seconds | −0.2 mph Ex: 6 | | | |
| (2 minutes) | 60 seconds | First start speed +0.4 mph Ex: 7.4 | | 0% | 1 minute walk/jog |
| | 30 seconds | −1 mph Ex: 6.4 | | | |
| | 30 seconds | −0.4 mph Ex: 6 | | | |
| (2 minutes) | 60 seconds | First start speed +0.6 mph Ex: 7.6 | | 0% | 1 minute walk/jog |
| | 30 seconds | −1 mph Ex: 6.6 | | | |
| | 30 seconds | −0.6 mph Ex: 6 | | | |
| (2 minutes) | 60 seconds | First start speed +0.8 mph Ex: 7.8 | | 0% | 1 minute walk/jog |
| | 30 seconds | −1 mph Ex: 6.8 | | | |
| | 30 seconds | −0.8 mph Ex: 6 | | | |
| (2 minutes) | 60 seconds | First start speed +1 mph Ex: 8 | | 0% | Cool down |
| | 30 seconds | −1 mph Ex: 7 | | | |
| | 30 seconds | −1 mph Ex: 6 | | | |

# WEEK 1—Run 3

Date: _____

Start Speed: _____

PB Goal: _____

Average Recovery Speed: _____

Mileage: _____

Notes:

_____

_____

_____

_____

_____

_____

_____

_____

_____

_____

_____

_____

_____

_____

# WEEK 2

Congratulations, you've made it past week 1! You will continue to learn some important foundations this week, in particular the importance of an active recovery. I also included a run in this week that requires a little more intense focus on your timing skills.

## RUN 4—RECOVERY ROAD

To start off this week we are going to have a unique and important lesson on the value of active recovery. We will do three rounds of six 60-second intervals. In each round we will find a new way to challenge our recoveries. The unique element of this run is that we will never increase workload on the actual interval, but we will on the recoveries.

# WEEK 2—Run 4

### Segment 1

*How To:* Your interval speed will remain **1 mph under your PB** the entire time. Your recoveries are going to grow rather steep. Note that the inclines are *only* on the recoveries, so after the interval you must add the said incline immediately. Also, try to keep the same walk/jog recovery speed each time.

| Interval | Speed | Your Speed | Incline | Recovery |
|----------|-------|------------|---------|----------|
| 60 seconds | Med./Fast Ex: 7 | | Int. 0%; Rec. 6% | 90 sec. walk/jog + 6% |
| 60 seconds | Same speed | | Int. 0%; Rec. 7% | Same + 7% |
| 60 seconds | Same speed | | Int. 0%; Rec. 8% | Same + 8% |
| 60 seconds | Same speed | | Int. 0%; Rec. 9% | Same + 9% |
| 60 seconds | Same speed | | Int. 0%; Rec. 10% | Same + 10% |
| 60 seconds | Same speed | | Int. 0%; Rec. 10% | 2–3 minutes complete recovery |

### Segment 2

*How To:* Now we will keep incline on 0% but challenge our recovery by making it shorter. Try to use the same recovery speed you used in segment 1 and react quickly on the last few, as a 40- or 30-second recovery is barely enough time to slow down and speed back up. That is part of the challenge.

| Interval | Speed | Your Speed | Incline | Recovery (all 0%) |
|---|---|---|---|---|
| 60 seconds | Med./Fast Ex: 7 | | 0% | 70 seconds walk/jog |
| 60 seconds | Same speed | | 0% | 60 seconds walk/jog |
| 60 seconds | Same speed | | 0% | 50 seconds walk/jog |
| 60 seconds | Same speed | | 0% | 40 seconds walk/jog |
| 60 seconds | Same speed | | 0% | 30 seconds walk/jog |
| 60 seconds | Same speed | | 0% | 2–3 minutes complete recovery |

## Segment 3

*How To:* Finally we will experience the third way to challenge your recovery: by making it faster. On this segment, choose an *exact* recovery speed that is 3 mph under your interval speed. From there you will be adding 0.5 mph to each recovery speed. Fill in your recovery speed column so you don't lose track. Note: if your interval speed is 6 mph or lower, I recommend choosing a recovery speed that is −2 mph instead of −3 mph, and you will simply add 0.2 each recovery instead of 0.5. That will ensure everyone is challenged regardless of ability.

| Interval | Speed | Your Speed | Incline | Recovery (all 0%) | Your Recovery Speed |
|----------|-------|------------|---------|-------------------|---------------------|
| 60 seconds | Med./Fast Ex: 7 | | 0% | 1 min. (−3 mph from interval) Ex: 4 | |
| 60 seconds | Same speed | | 0% | 1 min. +0.5 mph Ex: 4.5 | |
| 60 seconds | Same speed | | 0% | 1 min. +0.5 mph Ex: 5 | |
| 60 seconds | Same speed | | 0% | 1 min. +0.5 mph Ex: 5.5 | |
| 60 seconds | Same speed | | 0% | 1 min. +0.5 mph Ex: 6 | |
| 60 seconds | Same speed | | 0% | Cool down | |

# WEEK 2—Run 4

Date: _____

Start Speed: _____

PB Goal: _____

Average Recovery Speed: _____

Mileage: _____

Notes:

_____

_____

_____

_____

_____

_____

_____

_____

_____

_____

_____

_____

_____

# WEEK 2

## RUN 5—BLINK

To balance the challenging work done on the recoveries of the previous run, you are now going to be set free to do some short and fast intervals. This is a three-segment run, each made up entirely of 1-minute intervals. Within every interval there will be one or two changes of effort. Having those changes happen in such a short interval requires you to be very focused on the timing. These quick changes also are what make the run fun and engaging. React fast, and don't blink, or you may just miss a change.

### Segment 1

*How To:* Start **1 mph under your 1-minute PB**. On this first set of 1-minute intervals we will get good and warm with some incline bursts. Every interval is the same speed, but around the 30-second mark you'll add an increasing incline, finishing on a 20-second hill.

| Interval | | Speed | Your Speed | Incline | Recovery (all 0%) |
|---|---|---|---|---|---|
| (60 seconds) | 40 seconds | −1 mph from PB  Ex: 7 | | 0% | 1 minute walk/jog |
| | 20 seconds +% | | | 4% | |
| (60 seconds) | 40 seconds | Same speed | | 0% | 1 minute walk/jog |
| | 20 seconds +% | | | 5% | |
| (60 seconds) | 40 seconds | Same speed | | 0% | 1 minute walk/jog |
| | 20 seconds +% | | | 6% | |
| (60 seconds) | 40 seconds | Same speed | | 0% | 1 minute walk/jog |
| | 20 seconds +% | | | 7% | |
| (60 seconds) | 40 seconds | Same speed | | 0% | 2–3 minutes complete recovery |
| | 20 seconds +% | | | 8% | |

*THE ULTIMATE TREADMILL WORKOUT*

## Segment 2

*How To:* Start **on the same speed as segment 1**. Now, every interval starts with your starting speed, but then at 40 seconds you will add increasing speed for a 20-second burst of speed. There is also a decreasing incline to keep up the challenge.

| Interval | | Speed | Your Speed | Incline | Recovery (all 0%) |
|---|---|---|---|---|---|
| (60 seconds) | 40 seconds | Seg. 1 speed Ex: 7 | | 4% | 1 minute walk/jog |
| | 20 seconds +mph | +0.2 mph Ex: 7.2 | | | |
| (60 seconds) | 40 seconds | Seg. 1 speed Ex: 7 | | 3% | 1 minute walk/jog |
| | 20 seconds +mph | +0.4 mph Ex: 7.4 | | | |
| (60 seconds) | 40 seconds | Seg. 1 speed Ex: 7 | | 2% | 1 minute walk/jog |
| | 20 seconds +mph | +0.6 mph Ex: 7.6 | | | |
| (60 seconds) | 40 seconds | Seg. 1 speed Ex: 7 | | 1% | 1 minute walk/jog |
| | 20 seconds +mph | +0.8 mph Ex: 7.8 | | | |
| (60 seconds) | 40 seconds | Seg. 1 speed Ex: 7 | | 0% | 2–3 minutes complete recovery |
| | 20 seconds +mph | +1 mph Ex: 8 | | | |

### Segment 3

*How To:* Start **0.2 mph faster than you started segment 2**. Finally, we will aim to build our top speed not for the last 20 seconds, but for the entire 1-minute interval. We won't add speed on the last 20 seconds, but instead we'll add an incline of 5%. Note: because incline takes time to adjust, be sure to start adding the incline around the 30-second mark, to keep things honest.

| Interval | | Speed | Your Speed | Incline | Recovery (all 0%) |
|---|---|---|---|---|---|
| (60 seconds) | 40 seconds | Seg. 1 speed +0.2 mph Ex: 7.2 | | 0% | 1 minute walk/jog |
| | 20 seconds +% | | | 5% | |
| (60 seconds) | 40 seconds | Last speed +0.2 mph Ex: 7.4 | | 0% | 1 minute walk/jog |
| | 20 seconds +% | | | 5% | |
| (60 seconds) | 40 seconds | Last speed +0.2 mph Ex 7.6 | | 0% | 1 minute walk/jog |
| | 20 seconds +% | | | 5% | |
| (60 seconds) | 40 seconds | Last speed +0.2 mph Ex: 7.8 | | 0% | 1 minute walk/jog |
| | 20 seconds +% | | | 5% | |
| (60 seconds) | 40 seconds | Last speed +0.2 mph Ex: 8 | | 0% | Cool down |
| | 20 seconds +% | | | 5% | |

# WEEK 2—Run 5

Date: _____

Start Speed: _____

PB Goal: _____

Average Recovery Speed: _____

Mileage: _____

Notes:

_____

_____

_____

_____

_____

_____

_____

_____

_____

_____

_____

_____

_____

_____

# WEEK 2

## RUN 6—THE EVIL TWIN

This is one of my most popular formats! The concept of this run is to achieve a particular speed on one interval, and then repeat that speed but with a nasty little incline, the evil twin. It's a pretty easy format to follow, knowing that every flat interval will be paired with its evil twin.

## Segment 1

*How To:* Start **1 mph under your PB**. Begin with a pair of 60-second twins. You'll add 0.5 to the first twin, then incline on that speed for the evil twin. Note you will exceed your PB but only because you end on intervals less than 1 minute.

| Interval | Speed | Your Speed | Incline | Recovery (all 0%) |
|---|---|---|---|---|
| 60 seconds | −1 mph from PB Ex: 7 | | 0% | 1 minute walk/jog |
| 60 seconds | Same speed | | 8% | 1 minute walk/jog |
| 50 seconds | +0.5 mph Ex: 7.5 | | 0% | 1 minute walk/jog |
| 50 seconds | Same speed | | 7% | 1 minute walk/jog |
| 40 seconds | +0.5 mph Ex: 8 | | 0% | 1 minute walk/jog |
| 40 seconds | Same speed | | 6% | 1 minute walk/jog |
| 30 seconds | +0.5 mph Ex: 8.5 | | 0% | 1 minute walk/jog |
| 30 seconds | Same speed | | 5% | 2–3 minutes complete recovery |

### Segment 2

*How To:* Now we **start 0.5 mph faster than the end of the last segment**. That is the only speed change. You'll hold that speed on each set of twins as they get longer and incline goes down. You will really be asked to extend your elevated PB on the last few intervals, but you can do it!

| Interval | Speed | Your Speed | Incline | Recovery (all 0%) |
|----------|-------|-----------|---------|-------------------|
| 30 seconds | Last speed +0.5 mph Ex: 9 | | 0% | 1 minute walk/jog |
| 30 seconds | Same speed | | 4% | 1 minute walk/jog |
| 40 seconds | Same speed | | 0% | 1 minute walk/jog |
| 40 seconds | Same speed | | 3% | 1 minute walk/jog |
| 50 seconds | Same speed | | 0% | 1 minute walk/jog |
| 50 seconds | Same speed | | 2% | 1 minute walk/jog |
| 60 seconds | Same speed | | 0% | 1 minute walk/jog |
| 60 seconds | Same speed | | 1% | Cool down |

Date: _____

Start Speed: _____

PB Goal: _____

Average Recovery Speed: _____

Mileage: _____

Notes:

_____

_____

_____

_____

_____

_____

_____

_____

_____

_____

_____

_____

_____

# WEEK 3

You have now reached the halfway point and should be feeling a little more confident with your timing. Week 3 contains great variation between three very different types of interval workouts, experiencing a pyramid run, a fartlek run, and a repeats run. These are common workout styles in many running programs and refer primarily to the timing of the interval.

## RUN 7—HEAVY BASE

This three-segment run is actually a pyramid run, but starts and ends with a heavy base of 60-second repeats.

## Segment 1

*How To:* Start **2 mph under your 1-minute PB**. Very simply, you will add 0.5 mph to each of the four intervals here. You'll end just under your PB.

| Interval | Speed | Your Speed | Incline | Recovery (all 0%) |
|---|---|---|---|---|
| 60 seconds | −2 mph from PB Ex: 6 | | 0% | 1 minute walk/jog |
| 60 seconds | +0.5 mph Ex: 6.5 | | 0% | 1 minute walk/jog |
| 60 seconds | +0.5 mph Ex: 7 | | 0% | 1 minute walk/jog |
| 60 seconds | +0.5 mph Ex: 7.5 | | 0% | 2–3 minutes complete recovery |

## Segment 2

*How To:* Start with the **ending speed from segment 1**. You'll rise up the pyramid to a 90-second interval, holding the same speed on all intervals. You will also come back down in this segment, still holding speed, but starting to add the incline of the run.

| Interval | Speed | Your Speed | Incline | Recovery (all 0%) |
|----------|-------|-----------|---------|-------------------|
| 70 seconds | Last speed Ex: 7.5 | | 0% | 1 minute walk/jog |
| 80 seconds | Same speed | | 0% | 1 minute walk/jog |
| 90 seconds | Same speed | | 0% | 1 minute walk/jog |
| 80 seconds | Same speed | | 1% | 1 minute walk/jog |
| 70 seconds | Same speed | | 2% | 2–3 minutes complete recovery |

## Segment 3

*How To:* Again, you'll use the **same speed from segment 2**. Now you are back to the heavy base of four 60-second intervals but will finish adding incline. Notice we will end above the 5% incline rule, but I have set you up to be under your PB by 0.5 mph. It is modified for your safety and success.

| Interval | Speed | Your Speed | Incline | Recovery (all 0%) |
|----------|-------|-----------|---------|-------------------|
| 60 seconds | Last speed Ex: 7.5 | | 3% | 1 minute walk/jog |
| 60 seconds | Same speed | | 4% | 1 minute walk/jog |
| 60 seconds | Same speed | | 5% | 1 minute walk/jog |
| 60 seconds | Same speed | | 6% | Cool down |

# WEEK 3—Run 7

Date: _____

Start Speed: _____

PB Goal: _____

Average Recovery Speed: _____

Mileage: _____

Notes:

_____

_____

_____

_____

_____

_____

_____

_____

_____

_____

_____

_____

_____

_____

# WEEK 3

## RUN 8—FAST FARTLEK

This is a three-segment fartlek, and you will only be changing elements on the Fast minutes. Remember that in a fartlek your Easy minute acts as your only recovery.

### Segment 1

*How To:* Start **3 mph under your 1-minute PB**. This will always be your Easy speed in this workout. Your Medium is 1 mph faster than that, and your Fast speed to start is just 1 mph above your Medium. In this round the only change in the Easy-Medium-Fast cycle is that the Fast minutes are on increasing inclines. Remember, **your Easy interval is your recovery period**.

| Interval | Speed | Your Speed | Incline | Recovery (0%) |
|---|---|---|---|---|
| 1 minute Easy | −3 mph from PB Ex: 5 | | 0% | None |
| 1 minute Medium | +1 mph Ex: 6 | | 0% | None |
| 1 minute Fast | +1 mph Ex: 7 | | 3% | None |
| 1 minute Easy | Same Easy Ex: 5 | | 0% | None |
| 1 minute Medium | Same Medium Ex: 6 | | 0% | None |
| 1 minute Fast | Same Fast Ex: 7 | | 4% | None |
| 1 minute Easy | Same Easy Ex: 5 | | 0% | None |
| 1 minute Medium | Same Medium Ex: 6 | | 0% | None |
| 1 minute Fast | Same Fast Ex: 7 | | 5% | None |
| 1 minute Easy | Same Easy Ex: 5 | | 0% | None |
| 1 minute Medium | Same Medium Ex: 6 | | 0% | None |
| 1 minute Fast | Same Fast Ex: 7 | | 6% | 2–3 minutes complete recovery |

THE ULTIMATE TREADMILL WORKOUT

# WEEK 3—Run 8

## Segment 2

*How To:* Start with the exact **same Easy speed from segment 1.** It is also the same Medium speed, but it is the Fast speed that will grow 1 mph total to hit your 1-minute PB. Write in your numbers, as the increases on the Fast minute are very specific. Remember, **your Easy interval is your recovery period.**

| Interval | Speed | Your Speed | Incline | Recovery (0%) |
|---|---|---|---|---|
| 1 minute Easy | Last Easy Ex: 5 | | 0% | None |
| 1 minute Medium | Last Medium Ex: 6 | | 0% | None |
| 1 minute Fast | Fast (Medium +1.4 mph) Ex: 7.4 | | 0% | None |
| 1 minute Easy | Last Easy Ex: 5 | | 0% | None |
| 1 minute Medium | Last Medium Ex: 6 | | 0% | None |
| 1 minute Fast | Fast (Medium +1.7 mph) Ex: 7.7 | | 0% | None |
| 1 minute Easy | Last Easy Ex: 5 | | 0% | None |
| 1 minute Medium | Last Medium Ex: 6 | | 0% | None |
| 1 minute Fast | Fast Medium (+1.9 mph) Ex: 7.9 | | 0% | None |
| 1 minute Easy | Last Easy Ex: 5 | | 0% | None |
| 1 minute Medium | Last Medium Ex: 6 | | 0% | None |
| 1 minute Fast | Fast (Medium +2 mph) Ex: 8 | | 0% | 2–3 minutes complete recovery |

### Segment 3

*How To:* Again you'll use the **same Easy and Medium speeds from segments 1 and 2, but the final Fast speed from segment 2**. In this final segment you will extend the Fast minute to a 70-, 80-, and 90-second PB finish. Remember, **your Easy interval is your recovery period**.

| Interval | Speed | Your Speed | Incline | Recovery (0%) |
|---|---|---|---|---|
| 1 minute Easy | Last Easy Ex: 5 | | 0% | None |
| 1 minute Medium | Last Medium Ex: 6 | | 0% | None |
| 70 seconds Fast | Last Fast Ex: 8 | | 0% | None |
| 1 minute Easy | Same Easy Ex: 5 | | 0% | None |
| 1 minute Medium | Same Medium Ex: 6 | | 0% | None |
| 80 seconds Fast | Same Fast Ex: 8 | | 0% | None |
| 1 minute Easy | Same Easy Ex: 5 | | 0% | None |
| 1 minute Medium | Same Medium Ex: 6 | | 0% | None |
| 90 seconds Fast | Same Fast Ex: 8 | | 0% | Cool down |

# WEEK 3—Run 8

Date: _____

Start Speed: _____

PB Goal: _____

Average Recovery Speed: _____

Mileage: _____

Notes:

_____

_____

_____

_____

_____

_____

_____

_____

_____

_____

_____

_____

_____

_____

# WEEK 3

## RUN 9—LOAD AND FIRE

This two-segment run is a great blend of speed work and endurance. In each round we will gradually load up on speed within an interval, then we will use that speed on another interval plus incline. Load up the interval, then fire away for the entire length of the next interval.

## Segment 1

*How To:* Start **2 mph under your 1-minute PB**. This first segment contains six 90-second intervals. We start by "loading" up speed every 30 seconds of the first interval. Then we use that total added on the next interval but additionally "load" up on incline! You'll just miss your top speed in this round, but don't worry; it's coming for you in the next segment.

| Interval | | Speed | Your Speed | Incline | Recovery (all 0%) |
|---|---|---|---|---|---|
| (90 seconds) | 30 seconds | −2 mph from PB Ex: 6 | | 0% | 90 seconds walk/jog |
| | 30 seconds | +0.3 mph Ex: 6.3 | | 0% | |
| | 30 seconds | +0.3 mph Ex: 6.6 | | 0% | |
| (90 seconds) | 30 seconds | Last speed Ex: 6.6 | | 1% | 90 seconds walk/jog |
| | 30 seconds | | | 2% | |
| | 30 seconds | | | 3% | |
| (90 seconds) | 30 seconds | Last speed Ex: 6.6 | | 0% | 90 seconds walk/jog |
| | 30 seconds | +0.3 mph Ex: 6.9 | | 0% | |
| | 30 seconds | +0.3 mph Ex: 7.2 | | 0% | |
| (90 seconds) | 30 seconds | Last speed Ex: 7.2 | | 1% | 90 seconds walk/jog |
| | 30 seconds | | | 2% | |
| | 30 seconds | | | 3% | |
| (90 seconds) | 30 seconds | Last speed Ex: 7.2 | | 0% | 90 seconds walk/jog |
| | 30 seconds | +0.3 mph Ex: 7.5 | | 0% | |
| | 30 seconds | +0.3 mph Ex: 7.8 | | 0% | |
| (90 seconds) | 30 seconds | Last speed Ex: 7.8 | | 1% | 2–3 minutes complete recovery |
| | 30 seconds | | | 2% | |
| | 30 seconds | | | 3% | |

### Segment 2

*How To:* Start **0.5 mph faster than you started segment 1**. We will now do a smaller version of segment 1. There will be only one load of speed, so it will be a bigger jump. Your final interval will load up your PB speed on top of incline, and fire away.

| Interval | | Speed | Your Speed | Incline | Recovery (all 0%) |
|---|---|---|---|---|---|
| (60 seconds) | 30 seconds | −1.5 mph from PB Ex: 6.5 | | 0% | 1 minute walk/jog |
| | 30 seconds | +0.5 mph Ex: 7 | | 0% | |
| (60 seconds) | 30 seconds | Last speed Ex: 7 | | 2% | 1 minute walk/jog |
| | 30 seconds | | | 3% | |
| (60 seconds) | 30 seconds | Last speed Ex: 7 | | 0% | 1 minute walk/jog |
| | 30 seconds | +0.5 mph Ex: 7.5 | | 0% | |
| (60 seconds) | 30 seconds | Last speed Ex: 7.5 | | 2% | 1 minute walk/jog |
| | 30 seconds | | | 3% | |
| (60 seconds) | 30 seconds | Last speed Ex: 7.5 | | 0% | 1 minute walk/jog |
| | 30 seconds | +0.5 mph Ex: 8 | | 0% | |
| (60 seconds) | 30 seconds | Last speed Ex: 8 | | 2% | Cool down |
| | 30 seconds | | | 3% | |

Date: _____

Start Speed: _____

PB Goal: _____

Average Recovery Speed: _____

Mileage: _____

Notes:

_____

_____

_____

_____

_____

_____

_____

_____

_____

_____

_____

_____

_____

_____

# WEEK 4

As we head into week 4, the workouts are really going to start to grow in complexity and challenge. Be confident. You have prepared for this and are ready to take this next step toward your goals. When you get a little uncomfortable, remember, you made the ultimate choice to do this work. That rare commitment in today's world makes you exceptional. Go into this week knowing that this challenging work comes with a reward like no other!

## RUN 10—THE STRETCH

This workout shows you how to "stretch" challenging elements of a run. First you'll stretch out the duration of an incline, then a speed, and finally you'll stretch out both incline and speed for longer and longer periods of time.

# WEEK 4—Run 10

## Segment 1

*How To:* Start **2 mph under your 1-minute PB**. You will use this speed on every interval while taking on an incline after 30 seconds that stretches longer and longer up to a 60-second hill.

| Interval | Speed | Your Speed | Incline | Recovery (all 0%) |
|---|---|---|---|---|
| (40 seconds) 30 seconds | −2 mph from PB Ex: 6 | | 0% | 1 minute walk/jog |
| 10 seconds +% | | | 6% | |
| (50 seconds) 30 seconds | Same speed | | 0% | 1 minute walk/jog |
| 20 seconds +% | | | 6% | |
| (60 seconds) 30 seconds | Same speed | | 0% | 1 minute walk/jog |
| 30 seconds +% | | | 6% | |
| (70 seconds) 30 seconds | Same speed | | 0% | 1 minute walk/jog |
| 40 seconds +% | | | 6% | |
| (80 seconds) 30 seconds | Same speed | | 0% | 1 minute walk/jog |
| 50 seconds +% | | | 6% | |
| (90 seconds) 30 seconds | Same speed | | 0% | 2–3 minutes complete recovery |
| 60 seconds +% | | | 6% | |

## Segment 2

*How To:* Start all these intervals at the **same speed as in segment 1**. You'll follow the same format, but this time there is no incline and you'll stretch out a burst of speed up to a 60-second sprint.

| Interval | | Speed | Your Speed | Incline | Recovery (all 0%) |
|---|---|---|---|---|---|
| (40 seconds) | 30 seconds | Last speed Ex: 6 | | 0% | 1 minute walk/ jog |
| | 10 seconds +mph | +2 mph to max PB Ex: 8 | | | |
| (50 seconds) | 30 seconds | Start speed Ex: 6 | | 0% | 1 minute walk/ jog |
| | 20 seconds +mph | +2 mph to max PB Ex: 8 | | | |
| (60 seconds) | 30 seconds | Start speed Ex: 6 | | 0% | 1 minute walk/ jog |
| | 30 seconds +mph | +2.0 mph to max PB Ex: 8 | | | |
| (70 seconds) | 30 seconds | Start speed Ex: 6 | | 0% | 1 minute walk/ jog |
| | 40 seconds +mph | +2.0 mph to max PB Ex: 8 | | | |
| (80 seconds) | 30 seconds | Start speed Ex: 6 | | 0% | 1 minute walk/ jog |
| | 50 seconds +mph | +2.0 mph to max PB Ex: 8 | | | |
| (90 seconds) | 30 seconds | Start speed Ex: 6 | | 0% | 2–3 minutes complete recovery |
| | 60 seconds +mph | +2.0 mph to max PB Ex: 8 | | | |

THE ULTIMATE TREADMILL WORKOUT

## Segment 3

*How To:* Now you will combine some of segments 1 and 2. Again, start all these intervals at **the same speed as the other segments**. You'll then add a 3% incline and 1.5 mph each time and stretch that addition out longer over a 20-, 40-, and 60-second stretch. Keep in mind you now have to make *two* changes, so start adding incline a few seconds early, then bump your speed.

| Interval | | Speed | Your Speed | Incline | Recovery (all 0%) |
|---|---|---|---|---|---|
| (50 seconds) | 30 seconds | Last speed Ex: 6 | | 0% | 1 min. walk/jog |
| | 20 seconds +% & mph | +1.5 mph to max PB Ex: 7.5 | | 3% | |
| (70 seconds) | 30 seconds | Start speed Ex: 6 | | 0% | 1 min. walk/jog |
| | 40 seconds +% & mph | +1.5 mph to max PB Ex: 7.5 | | 3% | |
| (90 seconds) | 30 seconds | Start speed Ex: 6.0 | | 0% | Cool down |
| | 60 seconds +% & mph | +1.5 mph to max PB Ex: 7.5 | | 3% | |

# WEEK 4—Run 10

Date: _____

Start Speed: _____

PB Goal: _____

Average Recovery Speed: _____

Mileage: _____

Notes:

_____

_____

_____

_____

_____

_____

_____

_____

_____

_____

_____

_____

_____

# WEEK 4

## RUN 11—SHRINKING LADDER

This is a large three-segment run, focusing on shrinking a ladder of incline and duration while we increase speed. The intervals get shorter and the incline gets smaller, but you must balance the shrinking ladder with the perfect amount of speed increase.

## Segment 1

*How To:* Start **2 mph under your 1-minute PB**. This is the largest segment with the largest ladder. You will simply shrink the interval each time by 10 seconds and drop incline as noted. To balance that change, you will add 0.3 mph to each shrinking interval, so be sure to input those values in the Your Speed column.

| Interval | Speed | Your Speed | Incline | Recovery (all 0%) |
|---|---|---|---|---|
| 90 seconds | −2 from PB<br>Ex: 6 | | 6% | 1 minute walk/jog |
| 80 seconds | +0.2 mph<br>Ex: 6.2 | | 5% | 1 minute walk/jog |
| 70 seconds | +0.2 mph<br>Ex: 6.4 | | 4% | 1 minute walk/jog |
| 60 seconds | +0.2 mph<br>Ex: 6.6 | | 3% | 1 minute walk/jog |
| 50 seconds | +0.2 mph<br>Ex: 6.8 | | 2% | 1 minute walk/jog |
| 40 seconds | +0.2 mph<br>Ex: 7 | | 1% | 1 minute walk/jog |
| 30 seconds | +0.2 mph<br>Ex: 7.2 | | 0% | 2–3 minutes<br>complete recovery |

## Segment 2

*How To:* Start **on the same speed you ended with in segment 1**. This is exactly the format and concept of segment 1, except the ladder starts a little shorter and less steep.

| Interval | Speed | Your Speed | Incline | Recovery (all 0%) |
|----------|-------|------------|---------|-------------------|
| 80 seconds | Last speed Ex: 7.2 | | 5% | 1 minute walk/jog |
| 70 seconds | +0.2 mph Ex: 7.4 | | 4% | 1 minute walk/jog |
| 60 seconds | +0.2 mph Ex: 7.6 | | 3% | 1 minute walk/jog |
| 50 seconds | +0.2 mph Ex: 7.8 | | 2% | 1 minute walk/jog |
| 40 seconds | +0.2 mph Ex: 8 | | 1% | 1 minute walk/jog |
| 30 seconds | +0.2 mph Ex: 8.2 | | 0% | 2–3 minutes complete recovery |

### Segment 3

*How To:* Start **exactly on the speed you ended with in segment 2**. We will shrink the ladder one last time, and follow the concept of shrinking we did in the previous segments. Note: you will be asked to push the boundaries of your PB.

| Interval | Speed | Your Speed | Incline | Recovery (all 0%) |
|---|---|---|---|---|
| 70 seconds | Last speed Ex: 8.2 | | 4% | 1 minute walk/jog |
| 60 seconds | +0.2 mph Ex: 8.4 | | 3% | 1 minute walk/jog |
| 50 seconds | +0.2 mph Ex: 8.6 | | 2% | 1 minute walk/jog |
| 40 seconds | +0.2 mph Ex: 8.8 | | 1% | 1 minute walk/jog |
| 30 seconds | +0.2 mph Ex: 9 | | 0% | Cool down |

# WEEK 4—Run 11

Date: _____

Start Speed: _____

PB Goal: _____

Average Recovery Speed: _____

Mileage: _____

Notes:

_____

_____

_____

_____

_____

_____

_____

_____

_____

_____

_____

_____

_____

_____

# WEEK 4

## RUN 12—DOUBLE STUFFED

This is your Oreo run. You'll double stuff 90-second intervals with two 30-second intervals in the middle. We will work on incline first, then speed, then a combination of both.

### Segment 1

*How To:* Start **2 mph under your 1-minute PB**. This will be your only speed in this segment. You'll do 1% on all the 90-second intervals, and then inclines of 6% and 8% for the 30-second intervals.

| Interval | Speed | Your Speed | Incline | Recovery (all 0%) |
|----------|-------|-----------|---------|-------------------|
| 90 seconds | −2 from PB Ex: 6 | | 1% | 1 minute walk/jog |
| 30 seconds | Same speed | | 6% | 1 minute walk/jog |
| 30 seconds | Same speed | | 6% | 1 minute walk/jog |
| 90 seconds | Same speed | | 1% | 1 minute walk/jog |
| 30 seconds | Same speed | | 8% | 1 minute walk/jog |
| 30 seconds | Same speed | | 8% | 1 minute walk/jog |
| 90 seconds | Same speed | | 1% | 2–3 minutes complete recovery |

### Segment 2

*How To:* Start **1 mph faster than you started segment 1 (only 1 mph under your PB)**. That is your new 90-second interval speed. Your 30-second interval will grow 1 mph, then 2 mph, exceeding your PB (because it is for only 30 seconds).

| Interval | Speed | Your Speed | Incline | Recovery (all 0%) |
|---|---|---|---|---|
| 90 seconds | Last speed +1 mph Ex: 7 | | 0% | 1 minute walk/jog |
| 30 seconds | +1 mph Ex: 8 | | 0% | 1 minute walk/jog |
| 30 seconds | Same speed | | 0% | 1 minute walk/jog |
| 90 seconds | Last 90 speed Ex: 7 | | 0% | 1 minute walk/jog |
| 30 seconds | +2.0 mph Ex: 9 | | 0% | 1 minute walk/jog |
| 30 seconds | Same speed | | 0% | 1 minute walk/jog |
| 90 seconds | Last 90 speed Ex: 7 | | 0% | 2–3 minutes complete recovery |

## Segment 3

*How To:* Start **on the last 30-second speed from segment 2 (max)**. Now I really flip things on you. I switch the Double Stuffed, so that now there are two 90-second intervals stuffed between 30-second intervals. Your 90-second intervals are on a smaller incline and are **1.5 mph under your 30-second sprint (just under your PB)**. Look at the table closely and you'll see how it all works.

| Interval | Speed | Your Speed | Incline | Recovery (all 0%) |
|----------|-------|------------|---------|-------------------|
| 30 seconds | Last 30 speed Ex: 9 | | 4% | 1 minute walk/jog |
| 90 seconds | −1.5 mph Ex: 7.5 | | 2% | 1 minute walk/jog |
| 90 seconds | Same speed | | 2% | 1 minute walk/jog |
| 30 seconds | Last 30 speed Ex: 9 | | 4% | Cool down |

Date: _____

Start Speed: _____

PB Goal: _____

Average Recovery Speed: _____

Mileage: _____

Notes:

_____

_____

_____

_____

_____

_____

_____

_____

_____

_____

_____

_____

_____

_____

THE ULTIMATE TREADMILL WORKOUT

# WEEK 5

Now that you are really starting to master the flow of the runs, I'm going to start adding some runs that complement and relate to previous runs. Only 2 weeks to go. Make sure you aren't afraid to increase your Personal Best speed if you feel you've outgrown the PB you started using in week 1. Even elevating your PB from 7.5 to 8 mph will add a great new challenge and move you into a new level of running!

## RUN 13—HEAVY TOP

This is the opposite of the Heavy Base pyramid run. Now you'll have a "heavy top" once you climb all the way up your pyramid. There are three segments, with the top being the middle segment.

## Segment 1

*How To:* Start **2 mph under your 1-minute PB**. You'll start on a long 90-second interval and simply add 0.3 mph to each interval as they get shorter and toward the top. There is no incline in this segment.

| Interval | Speed | Your Speed | Incline | Recovery (all 0%) |
|---|---|---|---|---|
| 90 seconds | −2 mph from PB Ex: 6 | | 0% | 1 minute walk/jog |
| 80 seconds | +0.3 mph Ex: 6.3 | | 0% | 1 minute walk/jog |
| 70 seconds | +0.3 mph Ex: 6.6 | | 0% | 1 minute walk/jog |
| 60 seconds | +0.3 mph Ex: 6.9 | | 0% | 1 minute walk/jog |
| 50 seconds | +0.3 mph Ex: 7.2 | | 0% | 1 minute walk/jog |
| 40 seconds | +0.3 mph Ex: 7.5 | | 0% | 1 minute walk/jog |
| 30 seconds | +0.3 mph Ex: 7.8 | | 0% | 2–3 minutes complete recovery |

### Segment 2

*How To:* Start **on your end speed from segment 1**. You'll keep the same speed on each 30-second interval but climb to a 6% incline.

| Interval | Speed | Your Speed | Incline | Recovery (all 0%) |
|---|---|---|---|---|
| 30 seconds | Last speed Ex: 7.8 | | 1% | 1 minute walk/jog |
| 30 seconds | Same speed | | 2% | 1 minute walk/jog |
| 30 seconds | Same speed | | 3% | 1 minute walk/jog |
| 30 seconds | Same speed | | 4% | 1 minute walk/jog |
| 30 seconds | Same speed | | 5% | 1 minute walk/jog |
| 30 seconds | Same speed | | 6% | 2–3 minutes complete recovery |

## Segment 3

*How To:* Start **on your segment 2 speed**. Now you'll hold that speed back down the pyramid. Note: You will not hit your PB in this run, and you'll thank me for it on the 70, 80, and 90!

| Interval | Speed | Your Speed | Incline | Recovery (all 0%) |
|----------|-------|-----------|---------|-------------------|
| 30 seconds | Last speed Ex: 7.8 | | 0% | 1 minute walk/jog |
| 40 seconds | Same speed | | 0% | 1 minute walk/jog |
| 50 seconds | Same speed | | 0% | 1 minute walk/jog |
| 60 seconds | Same speed | | 0% | 1 minute walk/jog |
| 70 seconds | Same speed | | 0% | 1 minute walk/jog |
| 80 seconds | Same speed | | 0% | 1 minute walk/jog |
| 90 seconds | Same speed | | 0% | Cool down |

# WEEK 5—Run 13

Date: _____

Start Speed: _____

PB Goal: _____

Average Recovery Speed: _____

Mileage: _____

Notes:

_____

_____

_____

_____

_____

_____

_____

_____

_____

_____

_____

_____

_____

_____

_____

# WEEK 5

## RUN 14—THE SHIFT

This run is all about shifting gears on the final 30 seconds of each interval. There are only two segments in this run, one with longer 90-second intervals, and the other with 60-second intervals. You will really feel the workout leading into your final burst of speed.

# WEEK 5—Run 14

### Segment 1

*How To:* Start **1.5 mph under your 1-minute PB**. You'll do 60 seconds at that speed each time with an incline and then add 1 mph for the last 30 seconds with no incline.

| Interval | | Speed | Your Speed | Incline | Recovery (all 0%) |
|---|---|---|---|---|---|
| (90 seconds) | 60 seconds | −1.5 from PB Ex: 6.5 mph | | 2% | 1 minute walk/jog |
| | 30 seconds | +1 mph Ex: 7.5 | | 0% | |
| (90 seconds) | 60 seconds | Starting speed Ex: 6.5 mph | | 3% | 1 minute walk/jog |
| | 30 seconds | +1 mph Ex: 7.5 | | 0% | |
| (90 seconds) | 60 seconds | Starting speed Ex: 6.5 mph | | 4% | 1 minute walk/jog |
| | 30 seconds | +1 mph Ex: 7.5 | | 0% | |
| (90 seconds) | 60 seconds | Starting speed Ex: 6.5 mph | | 5% | 1 minute walk/jog |
| | 30 seconds | +1 mph Ex: 7.5 | | 0% | |
| (90 seconds) | 60 seconds | Starting speed Ex: 6.5 mph | | 6% | 2–3 minutes complete recovery |
| | 30 seconds | +1 mph Ex: 7.5 | | 0% | |

## Segment 2

*How To:* Start **at the same starting speed from segment 1**. You'll simply grow your starting speed each time by +0.3 to reach your PB as a starting speed. Halfway through the minute, however, I'm asking you to exceed your 1-minute PB, creating a new PB for the last 30 seconds of each interval. Whatever 30-second PB you set in the first interval will remain the number you try to hit in the last 30 seconds of all subsequent intervals.

| | Interval | Speed | Your Speed | Incline | Recovery (all 0%) |
|---|---|---|---|---|---|
| (60 seconds) | 30 seconds | Last speed Ex: 6.5 mph | | 0% | 1 minute walk/jog |
| | 30 seconds | Max +2 to 2.5 mph Ex: 8.5–9 | | 0% | |
| (60 seconds) | 30 seconds | Last speed +0.3 mph Ex: 6.8 | | 0% | 1 minute walk/jog |
| | 30 seconds | Top speed Ex: 8.5–9 | | 0% | |
| (60 seconds) | 30 seconds | Last speed +0.3 mph Ex: 7.1 | | 0% | 1 minute walk/jog |
| | 30 seconds | Top speed Ex: 8.5–9 | | 0% | |
| (60 seconds) | 30 seconds | Last speed +0.3 mph Ex: 7.4 | | 0% | 1 minute walk/jog |
| | 30 seconds | Top speed Ex: 8.5–9 | | 0% | |
| (60 seconds) | 30 seconds | Last speed +0.3 mph Ex: 7.7 | | 0% | 1 minute walk/jog |
| | 30 seconds | Top speed Ex: 8.5–9 | | 0% | |
| (60 seconds) | 30 seconds | Last speed +0.3 mph Ex: 8 | | 0% | Cool down |
| | 30 seconds | Top speed Ex: 8.5–9 | | 0% | |

# WEEK 5—Run 14

Date: _____

Start Speed: _____

PB Goal: _____

Average Recovery Speed: _____

Mileage: _____

Notes:

_____

_____

_____

_____

_____

_____

_____

_____

_____

_____

_____

_____

_____

# WEEK 5

## RUN 15—SWITCH BACK

This is a long and challenging run. You are ready for this. You will do a large interval, followed by a series of 1-minute intervals that grow in speed, then suddenly you'll switch back to the longer interval on its incline. This will continue in every segment but with shorter and shorter intervals.

## Segment 1

*How To:* Start **2 mph under your 1-minute PB**. This is a short segment, starting with the biggest interval on a 3% incline. You'll then add speed on a couple of flat 1-minute intervals, then switch back to the large interval on a 3% but of course on your elevated speed!

| Interval | Speed | Your Speed | Incline | Recovery (all 0%) |
|---|---|---|---|---|
| 2 minutes | −2 mph from PB Ex: 6 | | 3% | 1 minute walk/jog |
| 60 seconds | +0.2 mph Ex: 6.2 | | 0% | 1 minute walk/jog |
| 60 seconds | +0.2 mph Ex: 6.4 | | 0% | 1 minute walk/jog |
| 2 minutes | Same speed | | 3% | 2–3 minutes complete recovery |

## Segment 2

*How To:* Start **on your ending speed from segment 1**. This is a longer segment but follows the same format as the previous, starting with the biggest interval on a 4% incline this time. You'll then add speed on a couple of flat 1-minute intervals, then switch back to the large interval on a 4% with a new speed. You'll do this twice!

| Interval | Speed | Your Speed | Incline | Recovery (all 0%) |
|---|---|---|---|---|
| 90 seconds | Last speed Ex: 6.4 | | 4% | 1 minute walk/jog |
| 60 seconds | +0.2 mph Ex: 6.6 | | 0% | 1 minute walk/jog |
| 60 seconds | +0.2 mph Ex: 6.8 | | 0% | 1 minute walk/jog |
| 90 seconds | Same speed | | 4% | 1 minute walk/jog |
| 60 seconds | +0.2 mph Ex: 7 | | 0% | 1 minute walk/jog |
| 60 seconds | +0.2 mph Ex: 7.2 | | 0% | 1 minute walk/jog |
| 90 seconds | Same speed | | 4% | 2–3 minutes complete recovery |

### Segment 3

*How To:* Start **on your ending speed from segment 2**. This is the same format as the previous, but all the intervals now match. You'll do an incline on a 5%, then add speed on a couple of flat 1-minute intervals, then switch back to the 5% on your final speed. You'll do this twice and hit your PB on a 5% for your max challenge.

| Interval | Speed | Your Speed | Incline | Recovery (all 0%) |
|---|---|---|---|---|
| 60 seconds | Last speed Ex: 7.2 | | 5% | 1 minute walk/jog |
| 60 seconds | +0.2 mph Ex: 7.4 | | 0% | 1 minute walk/jog |
| 60 seconds | +0.2 mph Ex: 7.6 | | 0% | 1 minute walk/jog |
| 60 seconds | Same speed | | 5% | 1 minute walk/jog |
| 60 seconds | +0.2 mph Ex: 7.8 | | 0% | 1 minute walk/jog |
| 60 seconds | +0.2 mph Ex: 8 | | 0% | 1 minute walk/jog |
| 60 seconds | Same speed | | 5% | Cool down |

Date: _____

Start Speed: _____

PB Goal: _____

Average Recovery Speed: _____

Mileage: _____

Notes:

_____

_____

_____

_____

_____

_____

_____

_____

_____

_____

_____

_____

_____

_____

THE ULTIMATE TREADMILL WORKOUT

# WEEK 6

This is the homestretch! You've come so far and it's time to push through and break new ground in your fitness and running. This week is a combination of some of my all-time favorite runs.

## RUN 16—TRIPLE STUFFED

This is a play on the Double Stuffed run. This three-segment run will take you through a series of Triple Stuffed 60s. First you'll work on incline, then build speed, then combine both.

### Segment 1

*How To:* Start **3 mph under your 1-minute PB**. In this segment we will build up speed. Note: we won't hit your PB just yet!

| Interval | Speed | Your Speed | Incline | Recovery (all 0%) |
|---|---|---|---|---|
| 60 seconds | −3 mph from PB Ex: 5 | | 0% | 1 minute walk/jog |
| 30 seconds | +0.4 mph Ex: 5.4 | | 0% | 1 minute walk/jog |
| 30 seconds | +0.4 mph Ex: 5.8 | | 0% | 1 minute walk/jog |
| 30 seconds | +0.4 mph Ex: 6.2 | | 0% | 1 minute walk/jog |
| 60 seconds | Same speed | | 0% | 1 minute walk/jog |
| 30 seconds | +0.4 mph Ex: 6.6 | | 0% | 1 minute walk/jog |
| 30 seconds | +0.4 mph Ex: 7 | | 0% | 1 minute walk/jog |
| 30 seconds | +0.4 mph Ex: 7.4 | | 0% | 1 minute walk/jog |
| 60 seconds | Same speed | | 0% | 2–3 minutes complete recovery |

## Segment 2

*How To:* Start **at your ending speed from segment 1**. Follow the same format as segment 1, holding that speed, but now with incline increases.

| Interval | Speed | Your Speed | Incline | Recovery (all 0%) |
|---|---|---|---|---|
| 60 seconds | Last speed Ex: 7.4 | | 0% | 1 minute walk/jog |
| 30 seconds | Same speed | | 1% | 1 minute walk/jog |
| 30 seconds | Same speed | | 2% | 1 minute walk/jog |
| 30 seconds | Same speed | | 3% | 1 minute walk/jog |
| 60 seconds | Same speed | | 3% | 1 minute walk/jog |
| 30 seconds | Same speed | | 4% | 1 minute walk/jog |
| 30 seconds | Same speed | | 5% | 1 minute walk/jog |
| 30 seconds | Same speed | | 6% | 1 minute walk/jog |
| 60 seconds | Same speed | | 6% | 2–3 minutes complete recovery |

### Segment 3

*How To:* Start **at the same speed from segment 2**. Now you'll continue to add your last bit of speed to hit your PB. You must also do it on an incline!

| Interval | Speed | Your Speed | Incline | Recovery (all 0%) |
|---|---|---|---|---|
| 60 seconds | Last speed Ex: 7.4 | | 0% | 1 minute walk/jog |
| 30 seconds | +0.2 mph Ex: 7.6 | | 1% | 1 minute walk/jog |
| 30 seconds | +0.2 mph Ex: 7.8 | | 2% | 1 minute walk/jog |
| 30 seconds | +0.2 mph Ex: 8 | | 3% | 1 minute walk/jog |
| 60 seconds | Same speed | | 3% | Cool down |

# WEEK 6—Run 16

Date: _____

Start Speed: _____

PB Goal: _____

Average Recovery Speed: _____

Mileage: _____

Notes:

_____

_____

_____

_____

_____

_____

_____

_____

_____

_____

_____

_____

_____

_____

# WEEK 6

## RUN 17—SKYSCRAPER

Now we will build up an interval sky high! This three-segment workout takes you through building speed on a set of 1-minute intervals, then adding incline to those to make them 90 seconds, then adding additional speed to that to make it the ultimate 2-minute interval. The intervals will get challenging, so you are prescribed "matching" recoveries. If you feel you don't need the longer recoveries, still take them; just recover a bit faster. That's a good problem to have.

### Segment 1

*How To:* Start **2.5 mph under you 1-minute PB**. This is a short segment, with only four 60-second intervals. Simply add 0.5 mph to each interval.

| Interval | Speed | Your Speed | Incline | Recovery (all 0%) |
|---|---|---|---|---|
| 60 seconds | −2.5 mph from PB Ex: 5.5 | | 0% | 1 minute walk/jog |
| 60 seconds | +0.5 mph Ex: 6 | | 0% | 1 minute walk/jog |
| 60 seconds | +0.5 mph Ex: 6.5 | | 0% | 1 minute walk/jog |
| 60 seconds | +0.5 mph Ex: 7 | | 0% | 2–3 minutes complete recovery |

## Segment 2

*How To:* Start **on the ending speed from segment 1**. You'll essentially do the last interval from segment 1 but now building onto it an extra 30 seconds of 1–4% incline, creating a set of 90-second intervals.

| Interval | | Speed | Your Speed | Incline | Recovery (all 0%) |
|---|---|---|---|---|---|
| (90 seconds) | 60 seconds | Last speed Ex: 7 | | 0% | 90 seconds walk/jog |
| | 30 seconds +% | Same speed | | 1% | |
| (90 seconds) | 60 seconds | Same speed | | 0% | 90 seconds walk/jog |
| | 30 seconds +% | Same speed | | 2% | |
| (90 seconds) | 60 seconds | Same speed | | 0% | 90 seconds walk/jog |
| | 30 seconds +% | Same speed | | 3% | |
| (90 seconds) | 60 seconds | Same speed | | 0% | 2–3 minutes complete recovery |
| | 30 seconds +% | Same speed | | 4% | |

## Segment 3

*How To:* Start **on the same speed as segment 2**. You'll now do the last interval from segment 2 (90 seconds) but add on an additional 30 seconds of more speed, to create a mile-high 2-minute interval. Note: You will just barely exceed your PB. There are lots of changes in these intervals, so stay sharp.

| Interval | | Speed | Your Speed | Incline | Recovery (all 0%) |
|---|---|---|---|---|---|
| (2 minutes) | 60 seconds | Last speed Ex: 7 | | 0% | 2 minutes walk/jog |
| | 30 seconds +% | Same speed | | 4% | |
| | 30 seconds +mph | +0.3 mph Ex: 7.3 | | 4% | |
| (2 minutes) | 60 seconds | Start speed Ex: 7 | | 0% | 2 minutes walk/jog |
| | 30 seconds +% | Same speed | | 4% | |
| | 30 seconds +mph | +0.6 mph Ex: 7.6 | | 4% | |
| (2 minutes) | 60 seconds | Start speed Ex: 7 | | 0% | 2 minutes walk/jog |
| | 30 seconds +% | Same speed | | 4% | |
| | 30 seconds +mph | +0.9 mph Ex: 7.9 | | 4% | |
| (2 minutes) | 60 seconds | Start speed Ex: 7 | | 0% | Cool down |
| | 30 seconds +% | Same speed | | 4% | |
| | 30 seconds +mph | +1.2 mph Ex: 8.2 | | 4% | |

Date: _____

Start Speed: _____

PB Goal: _____

Average Recovery Speed: _____

Mileage: _____

Notes:

_____

_____

_____

_____

_____

_____

_____

_____

_____

_____

_____

_____

_____

_____

# WEEK 6

## RUN 18—TRIPLE CROWN

Who doesn't want to finish 6 weeks of workouts with a Triple Crown! This two-segment run will tackle all three ways to make an interval more challenging: by making it faster, steeper, and longer. Your ultimate challenge will be to combine all three challenges for the ultimate Triple Crown.

## Segment 1

*How To:* Start **2 mph under your 1-minute PB**. In this longer segment you will simply alternate between adding 0.3 mph to an interval, then doing that new speed on a 4% incline. You'll do eight 60-second intervals.

| Interval | Speed | Your Speed | Incline | Recovery (all 0%) |
|---|---|---|---|---|
| 60 seconds | −2 mph from PB Ex: 6 | | 0% | 1 minute walk/jog |
| 60 seconds | Same speed | | 4% | 1 minute walk/jog |
| 60 seconds | +0.3 mph Ex: 6.3 | | 0% | 1 minute walk/jog |
| 60 seconds | Same speed | | 4% | 1 minute walk/jog |
| 60 seconds | +0.3 mph Ex: 6.6 | | 0% | 1 minute walk/jog |
| 60 seconds | Same speed | | 4% | 1 minute walk/jog |
| 60 seconds | +0.3 mph Ex: 6.9 | | 0% | 1 minute walk/jog |
| 60 seconds | Same speed | | 4% | 2–3 minutes complete recovery |

## Segment 2

*How To:* Start **0.3 mph faster than your ending speed in segment 1**. You'll do that speed again on an incline, and a third time on the incline and longer. You'll do that cycle three times until you hit just under your PB, but for 90 seconds and on a 3%!

| Interval | Speed | Your Speed | Incline | Recovery (all 0%) |
|---|---|---|---|---|
| 60 seconds | Last speed +0.3 mph Ex: 7.2 | | 0% | 1 minute walk/jog |
| 60 seconds | Same speed | | 3% | 1 minute walk/jog |
| 70 seconds | Same speed | | 3% | 1 minute walk/jog |
| 60 seconds | +0.3 mph Ex: 7.5 | | 0% | 1 minute walk/jog |
| 60 seconds | Same speed | | 3% | 1 minute walk/jog |
| 80 seconds | Same speed | | 3% | 1 minute walk/jog |
| 60 seconds | +0.3 mph Ex: 7.8 | | 0% | 1 minute walk/jog |
| 60 seconds | Same speed | | 3% | 1 minute walk/jog |
| 90 seconds | Same speed | | 3% | Cool down |

# WEEK 6—Run 18

Date: _____

Start Speed: _____

PB Goal: _____

Average Recovery Speed: _____

Mileage: _____

Notes:

_____

_____

_____

_____

_____

_____

_____

_____

_____

_____

_____

_____

_____

_____

# DIET AND HEALTH

There are perhaps more diet books out there than any other health and wellness books. It's a tough subject to tackle in a workout book, but I do want to share some of the most useful eating and diet tips that have helped me in running and in keeping a consistently lean and strong body. I honestly believe that my commitment to running paired with my healthy eating habits have literally kept me the same weight and size for the last 12 years. I am 35, and I weigh exactly the same and have nearly the same measurements I had when I was 23—no kidding. That is the magic of running and eating healthy. Runners become fuel-efficient powerhouses! Here are some of the food strategies that have done amazing things for me.

## Tips and Tricks to Stay Healthy

### Water

This is number one. Most of us do not drink enough water, period. The first thing I do when I wake up in the morning is drink a glass of water, before I have a cup a coffee or eat anything. I try to make sure half my fluid intake every day is from simple, pure water. I recommend drinking 2.7–3.8 liters of water a day, which is about 13 cups. On days you do a run in this book, you have to make sure you are hydrated. Always sip water during these workouts, and make sure that you have been drinking water in the hours before. Coffee—I love coffee. In Michigan, I swear we are bottle-fed coffee! As long as you aren't overloading your system with caffeine all day, coffee is not only perfectly fine, but it's also a great natural energy booster before a run.

### Pre- and Post-Run Meals

If I am doing these workouts in the morning, I find I need to keep my pre-workout meal pretty light. These workouts are challenging, and you shouldn't have all your blood focused on digesting a heavy meal. When it comes to pre-run meals, think easy-to-digest. Foods like eggs, avocados, bananas, and oatmeal are great pre-run foods that will help keep your energy up and not weigh down the stomach.

An age-old trick for many runners is to consume citrus. Many athletes believe the citric acid hastens the reduction of lactate buildup after the workout. Lactate is produced during hard runs when oxygen intake can't keep up with the workload you are putting on the body. This lactate is used to break down glucose to help fuel your workout. The side effect of this, which is actually a clever defense mechanism, is to cause a slight burning sensation to prevent you from overworking or damaging muscles. One study, "Orange Juice Improved Lipid Profile and Blood Lactate of Overweight Middle-Aged Women Subjected to Aerobic Training," conducted in 2010, did in fact show that consuming orange juice dropped blood lactate levels by 27% compared to 17% in the control group. My go-to snack post-run is an orange, a red apple, or a banana. Keep in mind we all have different sensitivities, and some people find citric acid a bit "tangy for the tummy" after a run. I do feel a positive difference, however, and regardless of the amount of lactate flushing, the carbohydrate content of an orange or grapefruit is a fantastic fuel to replenish you as you recover.

### Fight the Free Radicals

Working out produces free radicals; there is no way around that. The good news is that these little radicals that can cause cell and skin damage can be battled. Here is an easy way to understand free radicals for those who are less than in love with chemistry. Free radicals are formed when a molecule sustains a broken bond and loses a critical electron. The molecule literally goes crazy trying to find its missing electron, and starts acting "radical" until it becomes a little thief, taking an electron from the closest molecule. It starts a chain reaction creating more free radicals, eventually leading to the possibility of cell damage. Hard exercise increases the occurrence of these free radicals, and so does long exposure to sun. Here is where antioxidants come in. We have all heard the antioxidant hype, and there is good reason for it. Antioxidants really do help fight free-radical buildup. The thing that makes antioxidants, like vitamins A and C, so awesome is that they can donate an electron to calm down a free radical, without turning into one themselves. They are stable with or without that donor electron. That is why it is important for you to have plenty of antioxidants in your diet. I do, however, warn you to be aware of where you are getting your antioxidants. Many juices and processed foods claim to have huge amounts of antioxidants, but the reality is most of them are damaged in the process and do not pack their full potential. With great conviction, I believe we must all get these antioxidants straight from the source. Another favorite snack post-run is a red apple, not green. I'm a huge fan of red and purple foods because of the massive amounts of flavanols, catechins, anthocyanins, and vitamin C that they contain. These are all powerful antioxidants. One of my favorite meals, once a week, is a purple cabbage salad with red berries, sliced red apples, and a mixture of seeds and nuts. Yummy, filling, and *so* good for you.

If I could recommend you research one more diet I would tell you to get a great book on the Mediterranean diet. It has been scientifically proven to be one of the healthiest diets in the world. I rely heavily on this diet, eating wild salmon, olive oil, and lots of protein from my vegetables.

Finally, cutting down on alcohol intake is one of the best decisions you'll ever make. You don't have to cut it out, but if you can cut it down, you won't believe how much it will change the way you feel and the way you look.

## KEY POINTS FROM APPENDIX A

- Stay hydrated; make it a priority.

- Avoid heavy, hard-to-digest meals before a run.

- Fruit is a great post-run snack.

- Be sure to get plenty of protein from your veggies.

- Include high-antioxidant foods in their raw and natural form. Bright and richly colored fruit and veggies pack a big anti-oxidant punch!

# TREADMILL TROUBLESHOOTING

While practice makes perfect, it doesn't mean you won't run into a few bumps along the way. Here are some tips on solving frequently asked questions and concerns.

## Timing—How can I better stay on top of the clock?

If you find yourself repeatedly falling behind on the clock, you may find success in writing down a running clock on your notes page or next to the interval column of each segment. So if your intervals are 70 seconds, 1-minute recovery, then 60-seconds interval, you can write:

> 0:00–1:10 (interval)
> 1:10–2:10 (recovery)
> 2:10–3:10 (interval)

### Speed—What if I discover my speed is too much or too little?

The built-in PB reference is there to keep this from happening, but we all have off days and really good days. If you feel you started too fast or too slow, simply adjust your speed down or up by +0.5 mph at any point in the run and continue with the instructed speed changes from that point.

### Incline—What if I need to modify inclines for medical reasons?

You should never modify inclines in the workouts because you don't "like" them. However, if you do have medical reasons for which you need to adjust incline, you can always create a smaller range of incline changes. For example: If you are asked to climb a 5–8% incline but have medical reasons for not going over 5%, you can adjust to go 3–5%. Incline modifications are reserved only for those with medical concerns or restrictions.

### Modifications for walkers and joggers—What if the starting speed feels too slow?

Commonly, those who max out at top speeds of 6 mph or less will feel the suggested amount to start below their PB too slow. If this is the case for you, you can simply cut the suggested amount below your PB in half. Then, when there are speed changes, simply add half the recommended amount and you'll tackle the same elevated workout as everyone else! Here is an example: If a workout says to **start 2.0 mph below your PB** and then **add 0.2 to each interval** after you start, you would instead start **1.0 mph below your PB** and then add **0.1 to each interval**. This will almost always solve the feeling of starting too slow, while still maintaining your PB.

## Mixing—Can I still take my favorite cycling class?

Yes, I want you to! I am not in the business of trying to take away the things you love. Cycling classes, yoga, weight conditioning classes, they are all important and you should mix them into the programmed workouts in this book. If you are cycling 5 days a week, however, you will need to cut back in order to successfully conquer the programs in this book.

Variety in your "non-running days" is so important. Going to the same studio, doing the same thing, day after day, no matter how fun it might be, is a mistake. I'm a running addict and I'm in the business of running, but even I make the choice to keep a balanced workout life. I struggle with yoga; it's frankly not my favorite thing to do. But I do it, every week, because I know it is good for me. I cycle, I swim, I weight train, and I take a killer rowing class all at the same gym. I may find running to be the most effective and my primary love, but these other variations keep me balanced, strong, flexible, and always learning. And that is important for a long and healthy life.

## I have a race—Can I still use the workouts in this book?

Absolutely! Although this book is not designed as a race training program, I have met countless runners who have told me that the exact workouts in this book have helped shave minutes off their racing times and achieve breakthroughs in their outdoor running. There are two successful ways to use the workouts in this book if you are racing outdoors. First, if you live in a climate where you normally miss quality months of outdoor running because of weather, these treadmill workouts will create a new foundation and preparation for when the frost finally does thaw. Second, the workouts in this book are great speed-work sessions toward the end of a training period for a longer race. Most distance programs have a tapper toward speed work leading up to the race, and many people have found great success in using these workouts for that period.

In addition, many first-time runners have used these workouts to gain stamina, strength, and confidence for their first 5k.

# ACKNOWLEDGMENTS

I would like to thank Jay Sures, Max Stubblefield, and Natasha Bolouki of United Talent Agency for seeing a greater potential in my voice and supporting the dreams and ambitions of my work. And to Caryn Karmatz Rudy at Diofore & Company and Brendan O'Neill at Adams Media for guiding me through my first book with such knowledge, patience, and grace. I must also thank Equinox for being true pioneers and leaders of health and wellness innovation and for their fierce support of their talent. They are the future.

I also want to acknowledge all the trainers and instructors who get up every day to change the lives of the people around them, but have not gotten to write a book or be on the cover of a magazine. I see you, I love you, and you matter more to this world than you could ever know.

And finally, this book is dedicated to Martin Richard, whose short but precious life ended at the 2013 Boston Marathon. I didn't know you, little man, but I think of you often as I tighten my laces. I will continue to carry your memory across the many finish lines of my life.

# ABOUT THE AUTHOR

**David Siik,** a native of Michigan's Upper Peninsula, is a graduate of Grand Valley State University in Biomedical Science and Chemistry, where he held multiple university records in track and field, including the 800-meter dash. Upon graduating, David spent six years in New York deepening his understanding of urban running while pursuing a successful career as a Ford model. Over the past decade David has become a well-recognized face in the world of sports and fitness advertising. He has been a contributing writer and been featured in publications such as *Men's Health, Men's Fitness, Women's Health, GQ, Esquire, Details, SELF, Shape,* and the *Huffington Post.* Most recently, David has been featured in the *New York Times* and the *Los Angeles Times,* on *Good Morning America,* and for the fifth time on the cover of *Runner's World* magazine.

David currently resides in Los Angeles and is the creator of Precision Running for Equinox, which has quickly become the industry leader in content-driven treadmill classes.

The uniqueness and precision of David's method combined with his enthusiastic and deeply compassionate approach to running have led him to become one of the most endearing coaches, motivational speakers, and educators in the re-energized running boom. His work has led him to be named by *Vogue* magazine as one of the "Best of LA." In the last year, *Details* magazine has featured David as one of the "hottest trainers to look out for," and *People* has applauded him with a full-page feature, naming him one of the leading innovators in fitness.